VOICE
PROBLEMS OF
CHILDREN

VOICE
PROBLEMS OF
CHILDREN

D. KENNETH WILSON, Ph.D.

Professor of Speech Pathology
State University of New York at Buffalo

The Williams and Wilkins Company
Baltimore 1972

Reprinted January 1973
Reprinted April 1974
Reprinted July 1975

Made in the United States of America

Library of Congress Catalog Card Number 70-178045
SBN 683-09060-7

Composed and printed at the
WAVERLY PRESS, INC.
Mt. Royal and Guilford Aves.
Baltimore, Md. 21202, U.S.A.

To
my wife
Frances Patton Wilson

CONTENTS

PREFACE

This book focuses on the voice problems of children. While its primary purpose is for use in training speech clinicians, it is also designed to be used by practicing speech clinicians in various schools, colleges, university clinics, hospitals, and the community as well as by clinicians in private practice. The contents will also acquaint physicians and other allied health professionals with the voice problems of children.

Pertinent material from diverse periodicals and books in speech pathology, medicine, dentistry, psychology, and education is an integral part of the text. The causes of voice problems are reviewed and examination procedures are described. Remedial methods and techniques are presented for voice problems due to laryngeal dysfunction and defects of resonance, and also those associated with hearing loss. The examination and remedial procedures are structured to be used as a practical guide for the speech clinician with emphasis placed upon the team approach to the remediation of voice problems. It has been necessary, in many instances, to adapt adult procedures to children since much of the available information on voice problems concerns adults. These adaptations were made as judiciously as possible and are primarily based upon clinical experience with children with voice problems. The need for more research and controlled studies of voice problems of children is therefore apparent.

The anatomy and physiology of the speech and hearing mechanisms have not been included in this book since comprehensive presentations are readily available in texts of medicine, dentistry, speech pathology, audiology, and speech and hearing science.

The voice therapy art illustrations were designed for special use by the speech clinician and were drawn so that the clinician himself can easily make facsimiles for use in therapy.

Thanks are due to many persons. Special thanks go to my wife, who was my chief advisor, researcher, and consultant; without her this book would not have been written. Special thanks are also due to my cousin, Geraldine Balsam, Art Instructor, The Packer Institute, Brooklyn, New York, for her voice therapy illustrations, and to Melford D. Diedrick, Medical Illustrator, The State University of New York at Buffalo School of Medicine, for his illustrations of laryngeal pathology. Thanks are also given to Ruth L. Powell, Medical Librarian, Veterans Administration Center, Bay Pines, Florida, Noretha Harper, Medical Librarian, Bay Front Medical Center, St. Petersburg, Florida, and Anthony R. Tusa, Interlibrary Loan Librarian, State University of New York at Buffalo, formerly at the University of Florida, for their help in obtaining reference materials. Special recognition is given to my parents, Dales and Gladys Wilson, for their interest and encouragement during the writing of this book, and to my daughter, Shannon, who as an active teenager often wondered when "quiet hours for book writing" would end.

D. Kenneth Wilson

Buffalo, New York

1

CHILDREN'S VOICE PROBLEMS

Children with voice disorders need comprehensive voice rehabilitation programs. The coordinated efforts of the speech clinician, parents, teachers, medical, dental, and health related professional personnel are necessary in these programs. Voice problems are identified, evaluated, and diagnosed, and then plans of therapy are formulated.

In order to evaluate a person's voice it is necessary to know the essential elements of a normal voice in contrast to the characteristics of a problem voice. A normal voice is essential for efficient speech communication. A good voice should have the following characteristics: (1) pleasing voice quality, (2) proper balance of oral and nasal resonance, (3) appropriate loudness, (4) an habitual pitch level suitable for age, size, and sex, and (5) appropriate voice inflections involving pitch and loudness. The rate of speaking should be such that it does not interfere with the five essential characteristics of a normal voice. This basic definition of a normal voice must be broad enough to allow a wide range of variation in any one or more of the essential positive characteristics.

To define a problem voice the five characteristics of a normal voice can be listed as negative characteristics making the answer to the question "What is a problem voice?" fall quite easily into place. A child has a voice problem if his voice shows one or more of the following characteristics: (1) laryngeal dysfunctioning causing disturbed laryngeal tone characterized by hoarseness, harshness, or breathiness, (2) improper balance of oral or nasal resonance causing hypernasality or hyponasality, (3) a voice too soft to be heard easily or so loud it is unpleasant, (4) an habitual pitch level too high or too low for age, size, and sex, and (5) inappropriate inflections of pitch and loudness. A problem voice may be distracting or unpleasant to the listener, and it may be severe enough to interfere with communication (1; 32).

Classification of Voice Problems

Voice problems are traditionally grouped into three categories: (1) pitch problems, (2) disorders of loudness, and (3) quality deviations. Deviations in rate in some instances are regarded as a fourth category of voice problem although rate is often classified as a problem of articulation or rhythm.

1

Van Riper and Irwin (40, pp. 272–273) pointed out while this is a convenient classification, "Seldom does the abnormal variation exist along one dimension of voice alone." A hoarse voice may be low in pitch or a breathy voice may be weak in intensity. This interdependence of characteristics makes classification of voice problems difficult. Thus we will define specific characteristics individually and then see how they are intertwined. Our definitions are based on subjective descriptions and on the results of acoustical analyses of defective voice.

Pitch Problems

A child has a deviation in pitch if his voice shows one or more of the following characteristics: (1) an habitual pitch level that is either too high or too low, (2) a very narrow pitch range, (3) too many pitch breaks, or (4) too high or too low pitch in specific situations. We are especially interested in a child's habitual fundamental pitch and whether it is appropriate for him. A too low pitch in an 8-year-old girl making her sound like an adolescent boy is as incongruous as a too high pitch in a 10-year-old boy which makes him sound like a kindergarten girl. We should also consider what the child, himself, thinks about his pitch level. One boy of 9 had what we considered a very high-pitched voice. However, the teacher and parents reported they thought his pitch level was all right but that he did not talk very much. Other children did not react to his high-pitched voice, and it did not seem to be a problem until we asked the boy himself what he thought about his voice. He replied, "I sound like a girl so I don't talk any more than I have to." Sadly he added, "You're a speech teacher can't you make me talk more like a boy?"

The high habitual pitch of childhood continuing in a boy after the usual age of voice change should be considered a serious voice deviation. During the period of voice change a boy's voice drops approximately an octave and a girl's voice 3 or 4 semitones. A child of 12 or 13 who uses higher pitch levels in his conversational speech does not stand out as being particularly different. However, when the child is about 14 or 15, whether a boy or girl, the voice change should be well under way. The speech clinician in a junior or senior high school should be especially cognizant of the period of voice change. If changes do not occur in a boy, or do occur in a girl to lower her fundamental pitch drastically, remedial measures should be considered. We recall one husky 17-year-old high school football player with a high-pitched voice. Examinations by the family physician, laryngologist, and psychologist revealed no organic or psychological basis for his high pitch. We were able to lower his pitch level approximately an octave during the initial therapy sessions and in about a month's time he was using the lower pitch level habitually in all situations.

Loudness Problems

A child may habitually talk so loudly that all the neighbors know his business and his family's also! He can easily be heard above the din of the school lunchroom, the teacher constantly tells him to talk quietly, and he is the loudest singer in the class. In contrast is the quiet talker who can never be heard. Everyone asks her to talk louder and to repeat until she gives up talking except when necessary. When she reads aloud in class no one can hear her so the teacher may think she has a reading problem. Often she is regarded as an extremely shy child. Her only problem may be that she does not talk loud enough. Results of various studies on loudness level vary according to the distance between the speaker and the sound measuring instrument. When measured with a sound level meter at about 40 inches without interfering background noise, loud talking is about 86 dB and soft talking about 46 dB (14, pp. 76–77). Draper, Ladefoged, and Whitteridge (11) agreed with this 40 dB difference between quiet talking and what they called "parade ground shouting." Black (5) found the range from soft to loud talking to be about 30 dB when measured 18 inches from a sound level meter, that is, from about 70 dB for soft speech to 100 dB for loud speech. He found a normal or natural level of loudness to be about 80 dB 18 inches from the sound level meter.

Voice Quality Problems

The third classification of voice deviations concerns quality of the voice. Voice quality problems include voices that are harsh, breathy, hoarse, hypernasal (excessive nasal resonance), hyponasal (inadequate nasal resonance), or with excessive glottal fry. There are two general types of quality disorders: (1) disorders of laryngeal tone, those associated with sound generated at the vocal cords, and (2) disorders related to resonance problems, hypernasality and hyponasality (27, p. 656). Harshness, breathiness, hoarseness, and habitual use of glottal fry are defects of tone generation. Sometimes hyponasality (13, p. 170) and hypernasality are considered articulation defects since they are related to poor use of the articulators. However, we classify hypernasality and hyponasality as voice problems since they are due to improper resonation.

Factors in Voice Quality

Before we specify the characteristics of voice quality problems it is necessary to consider the factors that make up voice quality. Voice quality is dependent upon four fundamental factors (37, pp. 209–210). (1) The basic structure of the vocal mechanism must be within the range of normal variation. Variations in structure of one or more parts of the vocal mechanism may account for differences in voice quality. (2) The physiology of the muscles and surfaces of the larynx, pharynx, nasal, and oral cavities must also be within the range of normal variation. If the muscles are tense or fatigued, if the surface tissues are abnormally dehydrated, if the surface tissues are covered with excess mucus, or if there is swelling or inflammation in any part of the vocal mechanism, the effects on voice quality will be deleterious. (3) Voice quality can be seriously affected by the individual's emotional status, either on a chronic or transient basis. (4) Voice quality is dependent upon good use of the vocal mechanism and may be affected by inadequate habits of voice production. Marge (25) studied speech and language of 143 children, 80 boys and 63 girls, nearly all of whom were in the sixth grade. Teachers and speech clinicians were requested to rate the children on 40 speech and language variables. As a result of a factor analysis voice quality was one of seven factors extracted. The variables which had high loadings for this one factor were quality of voice, articulation, appeal of voice, pronunciation, and flow of words. Thus basic to a pleasing voice is good articulation, correct pronunciation of words, and fluent speech.

Definitions of Voice Quality

Harshness. A harsh voice is unpleasant and rough (18, p. 209). Vocal fry may be present, considerable tension is localized in and about the larynx, and abrupt glottal attacks may be used frequently (39, p. 173). In an abrupt glottal attack the vocal cords adduct before the expiratory effort causing air to be impounded below the glottis. More pressure than normal must be applied to separate the cords resulting in the air being suddenly released with the voice sounding constricted and harsh (15). The harsh voice may be lower in pitch than is normal and also weak in intensity since many people find it difficult to obtain adequate loudness at low pitch levels (13, pp. 175–176). Bowler (8) found a mean fundamental frequency of 95.4 Hz for harsh voices compared to 127.1 Hz for normal adult male voices.

Breathiness. A breathy voice is characterized by whispered sounds and weak vocal cord tones (27, p. 656). The vocal cords do not fully approximate. This allows unvibrated air to escape between the cords adding a noise element to the voice (15). The vocal cords vibrate but because closure is not firm there is continuous air flow causing a person to have limited vocal intensity and low pitch (13, p. 179). A breathy voice may be mild or severe; in its mild form only a small amount of aspirate noise element is added, but in its most severe form all phonation is lost and we have only a whispered voice, that is aphonia.

Hoarseness. Hoarseness is quite common and occurs at some time in almost every person. It is at times overlooked and neglected by speech clinicians since it frequently accompanies and subsides with a common cold; thus there is a tendency to regard hoarseness as temporary and to feel the trouble will "clear up by tomorrow" (9). However, hoarseness is the unique symptom of laryngeal involvement and may be a significant complaint in many medical and surgical conditions (41). Hoarseness lasting longer than 10 days to 3 weeks should never be ignored (2; 30; 41). Its cause should be determined and removed when possible and voice therapy given when indicated. The term hoarseness is frequently used for any type of deviation of the laryngeal tone. However, the speech clinician should be able to distinguish a hoarse voice from a harsh or breathy voice.

Hoarseness in its simplest definition is a combination of harshness and breathiness with the harsh element predominating in some hoarse voices and the breathy element in others (13, pp. 182–183). Jackson (21, p. 576) described hoarseness as " . . . a quality of voice that is rough, grating, harsh, more or less discordant, and lower in pitch than normal for the individual." The hoarse voice has been the topic of laboratory studies. Moore and Thompson (28) analyzed ultra high speed motion pictures of the vocal cords and phonellograms of hoarse vocal sounds produced by two subjects. They concluded hoarseness is characterized by random fundamental frequency variability. Isshiki, Yanagihara, and Morimoto (20) found aperiodicity of the fundamental frequency present in hoarse voices with noise components and frequency variations in a voice closely related to each other. An increase of noise components in a voice will intensify the frequency variation. Yanagihara (44; 45) studied five vowels produced by 10 adults who had varying degrees of hoarseness—slight, moderate, and severe. Through spectrographic analysis he classified hoarseness according to the amount of noise present. He found that the range and energy of noise components vary with the perceived degree of hoarseness and are more evident in the vowels /ɑ/, /ɛ/, and /i/ than in the vowels /u/ and /ɔ/. He classified voices into four main types based on the presence of noise components in the different formants of these vowels. The types ranged from a small amount of added noise to almost complete replacement of the laryngeal tone by noise. Shipp and Huntington (36) rated and analyzed acute laryngitis in 15 adults with a mean age of 25.9 years, comparing the laryngitic stage to their normal voices after laryngitis had subsided. The fundamental pitch was the same under both conditions. The ratings indicated breathiness was related to hoarseness but harshness was not. They cautioned these findings may apply only to hoarseness accompanying acute laryngitis. Thus research has shown hoarseness to be related to breathiness, there is random fundamental frequency variation and aperiodicity of fundamental frequency in the hoarse voice, and noise components added to the laryngeal tone increase according to the amount of perceived hoarseness.

Hypernasality. Some nasal resonance is present in all speech. The /m/, /n/, and /ŋ/ are normally nasalized. When vowels are nasalized the quality becomes objectionable and is then called hypernasality. Hypernasality may also be present on consonants, especially consonants requiring a buildup of breath pressure within the oral cavity such as /s/, /k/, /ʃ/, /z/, and /g/. Sometimes these pressure consonants are nasally emitted with a characteristic snort. Assimilation hypernasality may be present when the vowels preceding or following /m/, /n/, and /ŋ/ are excessively nasalized because of their close proximity to the normally nasalized sounds.

A resonance problem may be the result of velopharyngeal dysfunction with or without an overt cleft palate. Hypernasality is not the best descriptive term for cleft palate type speech because often there is a peculiar combination of both hypernasality and hyponasality present. The speech of persons with imperfect velopharyngeal closure is characterized by excess nasal emission of sounds, hypernasality, and an inadequate oral breath stream with both voice quality and articulation often seriously defective (42).

Hyponasality. Hyponasality is a lack of nasal resonance on the /m/, /n/, and /ŋ/ sounds. The person sounds as if he has a cold and in the extreme form of hyponasality /b/ is substituted for /m/, /d/ for /n/, and /g/ for /ŋ/, resulting in word confusions such as *be* for *me*, *dew* for *new* and *rag* for *rang*.

Vocal Fry. Vocal fry (glottal fry) may be produced consciously by phonating quietly at the lowest possible pitch so the sound bubbles out of the larynx in discrete bursts (46, p. 197). Moore and von Leden (29) proposed the name dicrotic dysphonia for the voice quality commonly referred to as vocal fry; they established it as a physiological not a pathological entity. Vocal fry typically has a fundamental frequency below the average range of frequencies for a normally pitched voice. Timcke, von Leden, and Moore (38) found simulated vocal fry had a frequency of 75 Hz compared to the frequency of approximately 150 Hz before the change to the vocal fry. Hollien *et al.* (19) stated, "Vocal fry results from a train of discrete laryngeal excitations, or 'pulses,' of low frequency . . ." They stated that a reasonable frequency range for vocal fry is approximately 20 to 90 Hz. McGlone (24) found several subjects in his study had simulated vocal fry phonations below 20 Hz. He concluded the lower frequency limit for vocal fry may be at least an octave below that estimated by Hollien *et al.* He also found a very low rate of air flow associated with the production of vocal fry. We feel vocal fry can appear in harsh voices even when the habitual pitch is not particularly low. We have seen children with normal pitch levels who have an excessive amount of the popping cracking sound of vocal fry. Vocal fry in itself when present in a minor degree in the normal voice does not constitute a voice deviation; only when vocal fry is used exclusively is it considered a voice deviation (19).

Incidence of Voice Problems in Children

Many speech clinicians feel voice disorders in children are on the increase. Pressures of modern living and higher standards for school achievement are responsible for increased general tensions which result in vocal hyper-activity and a poor voice. Even so, some speech clinicians currently report that they have very few children with voice problems in their case loads. When asked to take a second look at children in their schools they find many more with voice problems. One school speech clinician who is very aware of vocal disturbances reported for the past several years that the incidence of all types of voice problems in his schools has averaged between 5 and 6 % of the school population with about half of them needing voice therapy on a regular basis and the remainder requiring attention from other specialists. Estimates and surveys of school children indicate that varying numbers of children have voice disorders. These estimates vary from 0.1 % to 2 %, indicating between 1 to 20 children per 1,000 with voice problems. In contrast actual survey results indicate many more children with voice problems.

Results of Voice Surveys

Results of voice surveys of children show approximately 6 % to 9 % with voice problems, which means between 60 to 90 children per 1,000. Pont (33) found 9.1 % of 639 kindergarten through eighth grade children with hoarse voices. Baynes (3) found 7.1 % of 1,012 first, third, and sixth grade children had chronically hoarse voices. James and Cooper (22) found 6.2 % of 718 third grade children had voice problems with about half of them having combined articulation and voice problems. Senturia and Wilson (35) reported 6 % of 32,500 school children had voice deviations. From these figures they estimated voice deviations occur in 3 million of the 50 million children in the United States in the age range 5 to 18 years. Assuming a more conservative estimate of 3 % with communicatively handicapping voice deviations Senturia and Wilson arrived at the figure of 1½ million children in the United States with voice problems.

Incidence in Case Loads of Speech Clinicians

Frick's (16) study is a good example of how many school children are receiving voice therapy compared to actual incidence. Fifty speech clinicians in Pennsylvania reported 2.01 % of the children in their case loads had voice problems but they estimated that the percentage should be higher. From their estimates Frick concluded the figure should be close to 5 %. Black (6, p. 7) reported in the state of Illinois public schools voice cases represented 4 % of the speech clinicians' case load. Voice problems represented 2.3 % of the case load of over 1,400 public school speech clinicians surveyed in a nationwide sampling (4).

Probably about half the children with voice deviations need voice therapy. The others have conditions requiring medical, surgical, psycho-logical, or psychiatric attention, and voice therapy is not indicated after successful treatment. However, those not needing voice therapy may involve the speech clinician in some way. For example in many instances it is the clinician's responsibility to see that children with voice problems are called to the attention of the proper specialists.

Identification of Voice Problems

Classroom teachers do not identify voice problems as such with accuracy. When a voice problem is combined with an articulation problem the accuracy of identification by teachers increases. Diehl and Stinnett (10) compared teacher referrals and the results of a school speech testing program of second grade children. Teachers were able to identify voice disorders with only 36.9 % accuracy while children with both articulation and voice disorders were identified with 70 % accuracy. James and Cooper (22) found about 10 % teacher referral accuracy with children who had voice disorders only. When the voice disorder was combined with an articulation problem teacher accuracy was about 52 %. White (43) noted voice problems in preadolescents and young adolescents are often overlooked since they are simply regarded as part of the maturation process. He felt these voice problems should be investigated and when possible eliminated. This avoids the development of an inadequate self image which together with the voice problem could later be handicapping both economically and socially. For example, an attractive high school girl who applies for a position as receptionist may be denied the position because of excessive hypernasality or a teenage boy may be ridiculed because of his high-pitched voice (26).

Parents generally are not concerned about voice deviations as long as they can understand their child's speech. They are primarily concerned about language development and clarity of articulation and pay little attention to the voice of their child unless it is quite defective. Either they dismiss the voice deviation as something the child will outgrow or they may not realize it is different. They may say, "His brother went through the same thing," or "Listen to the other children in the neighborhood." If they can understand the child's speech generally parents are not usually concerned about poor voice quality, deviations in pitch, or any other voice deviations.

The speech clinician should be aware of even minor voice problems. Some voice problems signal the possibility of actual physical problems or pathology. For example, a child with mild nasality may have a mild velopharyngeal insufficiency, in which case an adenoidectomy might create a severe velopharyngeal insufficiency with a severe voice problem. A child who has chronic mild hoarseness or a child with periodic hoarseness after periods of vocal misuse or vocal abuse may not be considered to have a problem. However, if he continues to use his voice in an improper fashion the hoarseness may become worse and result in pathological changes in the vocal cords. Any unexplained prolonged hoarseness indicates a need for immediate medical attention. Children needing voice therapy should have high priority in scheduling therapy. The speech clinician must see that all efforts are made to insure proper attention for all children with voice problems.

Vocal Rehabilitation

Children with voice problems require a careful appraisal of the problem, a detailed diagnosis, and a comprehensive treatment plan. These procedures require the joint efforts of many specialists from several areas, including speech pathology, audiology, clinical psychology, social work, dentistry, laryngology, pediatrics, otology, allergy, radiology, plastic surgery, neurology, and psychiatry. A child with a voice problem may first be seen by any one of these specialists. For example, a child with excessive nasality may be discovered in a survey by a school speech clinician or a child with a hoarse voice may be taken by his parents to the family physician or laryngologist. Children with voice problems often are first seen in community or college and university speech clinics. Referral and consultation with other specialists is usually necessary. A voice disorder in a child presents a challenge to those concerned. Many times the causes are unknown or obscure, the diagnosis requires time, and the rehabilitation takes even more time, effort, and patience. Appraisal includes a detailed description of the voice problem in all its aspects: laryngeal tone, loudness, pitch, and resonance. A complete case history is obtained. All the facts of the appraisal are gathered together and specific tests and examinations are selected to determine the cause or causes of the problem. The results of the tests and examinations are studied and the diagnosis made. The diagnosis is often difficult because the symptoms may be common to several different causes. For example, the causes of hypernasality include faulty learning, imitation, or a physical velopharyngeal insufficiency. It is necessary to differentiate these causes one from the other in order to find the basis of the hypernasality. A treatment plan is then devised and the prognosis or prediction of the amount of anticipated progress is formulated. The treatment plan may include medical, dental, and surgical procedures as well as psychological treatment and voice therapy.

The basic goals for the speech clinician in dealing with children with voice problems are as follows: (1) to aid in the prevention of voice problems, (2) to act as a member of a team of specialists contributing to appraisal and diagnosis, and (3) to offer a voice therapy program to modify or eliminate the voice problem. Prevention of voice disorders in children is an important function of the speech clinician. Many voice disorders of adults begin in childhood, especially in those children who go through much vocal strain including shouting, screaming, and singing in an unnatural range (12). Kallen (23) felt a planned school voice hygiene program should be instituted to save the voice from misuse and strain from the day a child enters kinder-

garten until he is well past puberty. Classroom teachers should be urged
to create an atmosphere in the classroom conducive to the development of
a good voice (34, p. 112). Froeschels (17) stressed the importance of good
vocal hygiene for children during reading instruction to prevent hyperfunction of the vocal apparatus. Special attention should be given to a
child who is hoarseness-prone. According to Boland (7) this is a person
who gets hoarse easily after sports activities, parties, colds, difficult work,
or emotional crises. The vocal behavior in a hoarseness-prone person is
characterized by excessive tension in the neck muscles with an inadequate
mouth opening for speech; this gives the impression of talking in the back
of the throat or down in the chest. A hoarseness-prone person may complain frequently of vocal fatigue and periodic hoarseness. The speech
clinician should discover children who are hoarseness-prone so they can
receive early consultation, appraisal, diagnosis, and treatment.

The speech clinician is an essential member of the team in contributing
to the appraisal and diagnosis of voice problems. He must be ready to
administer appropriate tests for the appraisal of voice problems and be
able to contribute his findings to the diagnosis. He should be prepared to
administer a thorough voice therapy regime. He must have an understanding of (1) anatomy and physiology, specifically of the speech and hearing
mechanisms, (2) the principles and basic methodology of learning, and
(3) the fundamental and specific methodology for the rehabilitation of
voice problems. We will concentrate on fundamental and specific methodol-
ogies for improving or correcting voice production. The results of selected
research studies with implications for appraisal, diagnosis, and voice
therapy for children will be reviewed. Many of the studies have been done
on adults and we will use some of the results as they may apply to children.
In summary, as Perkins (31, p. 835) stated, it is a goal of voice therapy
" . . . to train our patients to utilize their vocal equipment as hygienically
as possible so that they may speak extensively, forcefully, and effectively
without strain."

REFERENCES

1. ASHA Executive Council. The speech clinician's role in the public school. A
   statement by the American Speech and Hearing Association. *Asha*, **6**, 1964,
   189–191.
2. Barr, T. Hoarseness. *Texas State J. Med.*, **34**, 1938, 553–555.
3. Baynes, R. A. An incident study of chronic hoarseness among children. *J. Speech
   Hearing Dis.*, **31**, 1966, 172–176.
4. Bingham, D. S., Van Hattum, R. J., Faulk, M. E., and Taussig, E. Program organization and management. In Research Committee of the American Speech
   and Hearing Association, public school speech and hearing services. *J. Speech
   Hearing Dis.*, Monogr. Suppl. 8, 1961.
5. Black, J. W. Relationships among fundamental frequency, vocal sound pressure,
   and rate of speaking. *Lang. Speech*, **4**, 1961, 196–199.
6. Black, M. E. *Speech correction in the schools*. Englewood Cliffs: Prentice-Hall,
   Inc., 1964.

7. Boland, J. L., Jr. Voice therapy for hoarse voice. *J. Okla. Med. Ass.*, **46**, 1953, 109–113.
8. Bowler, N. W. A fundamental frequency analysis of harsh vocal quality. *Speech Monogr.*, **31**, 1964, 128–134.
9. Damitz, J. C., and Dill, J. L. Chronic hoarseness: Report of three hundred consecutive cases. *Ann. Otol.*, **49**, 1940, 996–1007.
10. Diehl, C. F., and Stinnett, C. D. Efficiency of teacher referrals in a school speech testing program. *J. Speech Hearing Dis.*, **24**, 1959, 34–36.
11. Draper, M. H., Ladefoged, P., and Whitteridge, D. Expiratory pressures and air flow during speech. *Brit. Med. J.*, **18**, 1960, 1837–1843.
12. Ellis, M. Remarks on dysphonia. *J. Laryng.*, **73**, 1959, 99–103.
13. Fairbanks, G. *Voice and articulation drillbook.* Ed. 2. New York: Harper and Brothers, 1960.
14. Fletcher, H. *Speech and hearing in communication.* Princeton: D. Van Nostrand Company, 1953.
15. Fomon, S., Bell, J. W., Lubart, J., Schattner, A., and Syracuse, V. R. Otolaryngology and speech therapy. *Eye, Ear, Nose, Throat Monthly*, **45**, 1966, 71, 72, 74, 76.
16. Frick, J. V. The incidence of voice defects among school-age speech defective children. *Penn. Speech Ann.*, **17**, 1960, 61–62.
17. Froeschels, E. Laws in the appearance and the development of voice hyperfunctions. *J. Speech Dis.*, **5**, 1940, 1–4.
18. Hanley, T. D., and Thurman, W. L. *Developing vocal skills.* Ed. 2. New York: Holt, Rinehart and Winston, Inc., 1970.
19. Hollien, H., Moore, P., Wendahl, R., and Michel, J. On the nature of vocal fry. *J. Speech Hearing Res.*, **9**, 1966, 245–247.
20. Isshiki, N., Yanagihara, N., and Morimoto, M. Approach to the objective diagnosis of hoarseness. *Folia Phoniat. (Basel)*, **18**, 1966, 393–400.
21. Jackson, C. Hoarseness. In C. Jackson and C. L. Jackson (Editors), *Diseases of the nose, throat, and ear.* Ed. 2. Philadelphia: W. B. Saunders Company, 1959.
22. James, H. P., and Cooper, E. B. Accuracy of teacher referrals of speech handicapped children. *Exceptional Child.*, **33**, 1966, 29–33.
23. Kallen, L. A. What is "optimal" for the human voice? *Logos*, **2**, 1959, 40–48.
24. McGlone, R. E. Air flow during vocal fry phonation. *J. Speech Hearing Res.*, **10**, 1967, 299–304.
25. Marge, M. A factor analysis of oral communication skills in older children. *J. Speech Hearing Res.*, **7**, 1964, 31–46.
26. Moore, M. V. Help for the child with a voice disorder. *Alabama School J.*, **84**, 1967, 30–31, 40, 42.
27. Moore, G. P. Voice disorders associated with organic abnormalities. In L. E. Travis (Editor), *Handbook of speech pathology.* New York: Appleton-Century-Crofts, Inc., 1957.
28. Moore, P., and Thompson, C. L. Comments on physiology of hoarseness. *Arch. Otolaryng. (Chicago)*, **81**, 1965, 97–102.
29. Moore, P., and von Leden, H. Dynamic variations of the vibratory pattern in the normal larynx. *Folia Phoniat. (Basel)*, **10**, 1958, 205–238.
30. Negus, V. E. The significance of hoarseness. *New York J. Med.*, **39**, 1939, 9–12.
31. Perkins, W. H. The challenge of functional disorders of voice. In L. E. Travis (Editor), *Handbook of speech pathology.* New York: Appleton-Century-Crofts, Inc., 1957.
32. Peterson, G. E. Influence of voice quality. *Volta Rev.*, **48**, 1946, 640–641.
33. Pont, C. Hoarseness in children. *W. Mich. Univ. J. Speech Ther.*, **2**, 1965, 6–8.
34. Pronovost, W., and Kingman, L. *The teaching of speaking and listening in the elementary school.* New York: Longmans, Green and Company, 1959.
35. Senturia, B. H., and Wilson, F. B. Otorhinolaryngic findings in children with voice deviations. *Ann. Otol.*, **77**, 1968, 1027–1041.
36. Shipp, T., and Huntington, D. A. Some acoustic and perceptual factors in acute laryngitic hoarseness. *J. Speech Hearing Dis.*, **30**, 1965, 350–359.

37. Strother, C. R. Voice improvement. In J. M. O'Neill (Editor), *Foundations of speech*. New York: Prentice-Hall, Inc., 1942.
38. Timcke, R., von Leden, H., and Moore, P. Laryngeal vibrations: Measurements of the glottic wave. Part II. Physiologic variations. *Arch. Otolaryng. (Chicago)*, **69**, 1959, 438–444.
39. Van Riper, C. *Speech correction. Principles and methods*. Ed. 4. Englewood Cliffs: Prentice-Hall, Inc., 1963.
40. Van Riper, C., and Irwin, J. V. *Voice and articulation*. Englewood Cliffs: Prentice-Hall, Inc., 1958.
41. von Leden, H. The clinical significance of hoarseness and related voice disorders. *J. Lancet*, **78**, 1958, 50–53.
42. Ward, P., and Wepman, J. M. Pharyngeal implants for reduction of air space in velopharyngeal insufficiency. I. An experimental study. *Ann. Otol.*, **73**, 1964, 443–457.
43. White, F. W. Some causes of hoarseness in children. *Ann. Otol.*, **55**, 1946, 537–542.
44. Yanagihara, N. Hoarseness: Investigations of the physiological mechanisms. *Ann. Otol.*, **76**, 1967, 472–488.
45. Yanagihara, N. Significance of harmonic changes and noise components in hoarseness. *J. Speech Hearing Res.*, **10**, 1967, 531–541.
46. Zemlin, W. R. *Speech and hearing science. Anatomy and physiology*. Englewood Cliffs: Prentice-Hall, Inc., 1968.

2

CAUSES OF VOICE PROBLEMS
IN CHILDREN

The causes of voice problems in children can be divided into four categories: (1) organic, (2) organic changes resulting from vocal abuse and vocal misuse, (3) functional, and (4) factors contributing to the voice problem.

The causes of voice problems exist on a continuum with organic at one end and functional at the other (86, p. 654; 90, p. 2; 115, pp. 321–322). Congenital or adventitiously acquired laryngeal, pharyngeal, oral, or nasal deviations lie at the organic end of the continuum. Voice problems due to emotional disturbances or poor voice standards in the environment lie at the functional end of the continuum. The continuum is a two way path because a pathology can result in a poorly functioning mechanism or a poorly functioning voice mechanism can result in organic changes or an organic condition (86, p. 654; 90, p. 2; 115, pp. 31–32). It is difficult to make a clear distinction between organic and functional voice problems; while some form of organic disease or structural anomaly is the primary cause in an organic voice disorder, some functional elements may be present (21, p. 47). Sometimes the psychological reaction to an organic problem causes a voice problem ". . . far in excess of the organic impairment" (21, p. 47). Every vocal deficiency has a psychic effect, whether it is conscious or unconscious, acknowledged or secret (118). A vocal dysfunction may continue long after the organic voice disorder becomes functional (21, p. 47; 115, p. 322).

Structural or pathological changes occurring as the result of faulty use of the vocal mechanism lie in the middle of the continuum. We label this cause "organic changes resulting from vocal abuse and vocal misuse." Brodnitz (22) stated patients who have developed an organic condition as a result of vocal abuse or misuse do not belong in the same category as patients with bona fide organic damage such as paralysis of a vocal cord. Our final classification includes factors such as allergies and upper respiratory diseases which contribute to the other three causes. All four types of causes may be so intertwined that determining the specific cause or causes of a voice problem may be difficult.

Organic Causes of Voice Problems

Some children have voice problems present on an organic basis. There are five sites of organic causes of voice disorders: the larynx, the velopharyngeal area, the oral cavity, the nose, and the hearing mechanism. Voice problems due to laryngeal involvements cause the voice to sound harsh, breathy, hoarse, or with inappropriate pitch; defects in the velopharyngeal area cause the voice to sound hypernasal, sometimes with a typical cleft palate type quality; defects of the palate and sometimes the tongue also cause hypernasality; and defects involving the nose usually result in hyponasal (denasal) voice quality. Hearing loss may affect loudness, pitch, resonance, laryngeal tone, and rate.

The Larynx

Organic causes of voice problems arising in the larynx and the immediate surrounding areas are as follows: (1) structural anomalies, (2) paralysis of any one or several of the nerves supplying the larynx, (3) growths in or around the larynx, and (4) trauma to the larynx.

Structural Anomalies. Structural anomalies may be present on a congenital or developmental basis. In some cases these anomalies can be treated by surgical operations. In selected cases voice therapy is indicated. Close attention should be paid to children with these types of problems as their voices develop to determine if voice therapy is needed. Let us look at specific structural anomalies.

Congenital laryngeal webs may be supraglottic, glottic, or subglottic; they generally involve the anterior portion of the glottis (73, p. 205) and consist of thin connective tissue. The ventricular bands also may be involved (7). Laryngeal webs may range from a small anterior commissure webbing to almost complete closure of the glottis (54) (Figs. 1 and 2). A complete web is incompatible with life and requires immediate surgical attention (34, p. 112). The symptoms of congenital laryngeal webs in the infant consist of hoarse, weak, or absent cry, and sometimes difficulty in breathing (58). The treatment of laryngeal web is in the hands of the physician and consists of excision or dilatation of the web (73, pp. 205–206). In some instances, after the web has been removed there may be vocal disturbances present sometimes manifested in a high-pitched and weak voice requiring voice therapy. The condition is not always diagnosed when the patient is an infant (58). A small anterior web may not interfere with breathing and its only influence may occur at the age of expected voice change. In this instance the high pitch of childhood continues because of the shortened vibrating portions of the vocal cords (87, p. 97). Teenage boys with high-pitched voices need a careful laryngeal examination to rule out the possibility of a web.

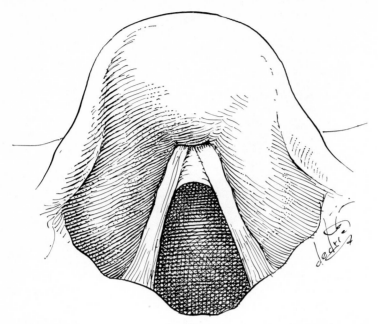

Fig. 1. Congenital web (small anterior). Illustration by Melford D. Diedrick.

Underdevelopment of one vocal cord may be present on a congenital or developmental basis resulting in an aspirate voice (130, pp. 220–221). The shape of the arytenoid and its attachment to the vocal cords may not be symmetrical (130, p. 221). In this condition also the child is likely to have an aspirate voice quality because of inadequate approximation of the vocal cords (130, p. 221).

Other congenital anomalies include absence of the epiglottis, deformities of the cricoid cartilage, and a laryngo-esophageal cleft (54). A few cases of congenital vascular anomalies of the larynx have been reported (54).

Some congenital laryngeal conditions are of interest to the speech clinician if voice problems develop as the child grows. These include congenital laryngeal stridor and congenital subglottic stenosis (54). Laryngomalacia (congenital laryngeal stridor) ordinarily disappears between the 12th and 18th month (54). It is caused by a failure of the cartilages of the larynx, especially the epiglottis, to develop normally; during inspiration the epiglottis and the aryepiglottic folds collapse into the airway (109) (Fig. 3). This results in a loud staccato repetitive crowing noise when the child inhales (54). Congenital subglottic stenosis may be severe enough to require surgical or medical treatment or it may be mild enough to disappear as the child matures (54).

Hyperkinetic dysphonia may be the result of a congenital structural

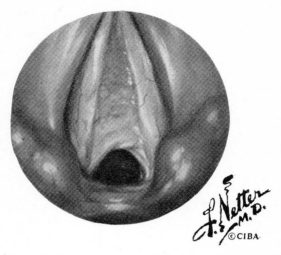

Fig. 2. Congenital web (incomplete) viewed through laryngoscope. Copyright *Clinical Symposia* by Frank H. Netter, M.D., published by CIBA Pharmaceutical Company.

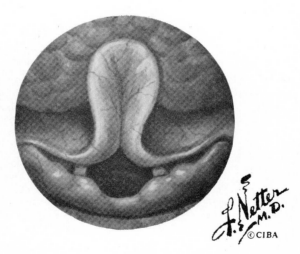

Fig. 3. Laryngomalacia (congenital laryngeal stridor). Copyright *Clinical Symposia* by Frank H. Netter, M.D., published by CIBA Pharmaceutical Company.

anomaly and was described by Luchsinger (80, pp. 303–306) as follows: "It is characterized by the excessive contraction of all muscles participating in phonation" including the laryngeal muscles, muscles of the respiratory apparatus, and the cervical suspension muscles of the larynx. The voice is harsh, strained, and sometimes muffled and sometimes overly loud. The child talks in this manner to overcome asymmetry or weakness of the laryngeal structure. The larynx shows the results of irritation in the form of hyperemia, swelling, and epithelial thickening of the vocal cord margins. Voice therapy is usually indicated.

Vocal Cord Paralysis. Vocal cord paralysis may be congenital or may appear as a result of trauma, growths, or illness. It may affect one or both vocal cords (54). The condition is more serious if both vocal cords are affected. The actual incidence is unknown, but it should be noted that this type of problem is not seen frequently in children (56). When it does appear in children the abductor muscles are the ones usually affected (73, p. 212). The paralysis may be either spastic or flaccid, but it is difficult to differentiate between them (34, p. 95). Typical vocal characteristics in laryngeal paralysis are hoarseness, a weak soft voice, and breathiness. Vocal characteristics are more deviant when both vocal cords are involved. Laryngeal paralysis is often accompanied by dyspnea or stridor (30; 34, p. 97). Cavanagh (30) presented a comprehensive study of vocal paralysis in 37 children examined by direct laryngoscopy. The onset of symptoms occurred in 11 of them at birth and in the remainder up to 7 years of age. She could determine the cause of the vocal palsy in only 8 of these children. Congenital paralysis of one or both vocal cords in an infant is often associated with other abnormalities (30; 54). Unilateral vocal cord paralysis in infants more frequently affects the left vocal cord (54). The prognosis for voice function with right cord paralysis is good, for those with left cord paralysis only fair, since the latter is often associated with anomalies of the heart and great blood vessels (54).

Laryngeal Growths. Growths or tumors in the laryngeal area are primarily a medical problem. They result in stenosis of the air passage and when they are enlarged may cause some degree of respiratory obstruction. Types of growths seen in children are papillomas, cysts, and laryngoceles.

Papilloma in and around the larynx may cause hoarseness and sometimes aphonia. Laryngeal papillomatosis is a serious debilitating clinical problem both in children and adults (55) and may involve air hunger and stridor (34, p. 125). A papilloma is a wartlike growth thought to be caused by a virus (34, pp. 124–125) (Figs. 4 and 5). Various methods of treating a child for papilloma are used, one of them being surgery; since they often recur repeated surgery is common (34, p. 125). Great care must be exercised in removing papilloma or permanent hoarseness may result if vocal cords are damaged (34, p. 125). Voice therapy usually is indicated when hoarseness persists after removal of the papilloma (57). Voice improvement is especially difficult in cases where surgery has resulted in a roughening of the free margins of the vocal cords.

Congenital cysts may have their origin in the vocal cords, the ventricle, or the aryepiglottic folds (7). They may be discovered at birth or during

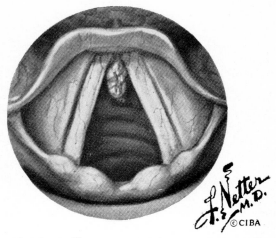

FIG. 4. Pedunculated papilloma at anterior commissure. Copyright *Clinical Symposia* by Frank H. Netter, M.D., published by CIBA Pharmaceutical Company.

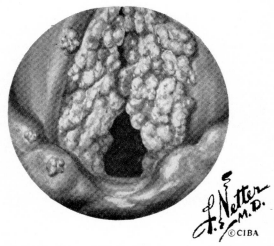

FIG. 5. Juvenile papillomatosis (laryngoscopic view). Copyright *Clinical Symposia* by Frank H. Netter, M.D., published by CIBA Pharmaceutical Company.

childhood; successful treatment is by operation to remove the cyst (7). The voice is usually adequate after an operation; however, at times voice therapy may be indicated to overcome laryngeal insufficiency resulting from the operation.

A congenital laryngocele may be difficult to distinguish from a cyst (54). It originates from the ventricle and is a sac filled either with air or fluid (54). It may bulge out between the true and false vocal cords (54). It may even be visible externally between the hyoid bone and the thyroid cartilage during coughing or straining (73, p. 210). The symptoms are hoarseness and dyspnea (58).

Malignant tumors as a cause of voice problems in children are rare (73, p. 208). There are reports of children who have undergone some form of therapy for cancer of the larynx, either partial removal of the larynx or total laryngectomy. However, these cases are so few that they are not of major concern to the speech clinician.

Laryngeal Trauma. Damage to the larynx may occur in children as a result of automobile accidents (57), inhaling toxic (59) or caustic (73, p. 208) substances, intubation either during operations or upon delivery (57), tracheotomy (73, p. 208), and aspiration of foreign objects (57; 73, p. 211). Injury may cause damage to either the joints or musculature of the larynx (5) or may result in fracture of laryngeal cartilages (57). Intubation may be necessary to relieve respiratory problems in an infant who has difficulty breathing upon delivery (57), or it may be done during an operation. Laryngotracheal complications which follow endotracheal intubation are inflammatory or allergic edema, ulceration of the laryngotracheal mucosa, laryngitis and tracheitis, glottic web, avulsion of a vocal cord (a forcible separation or detachment of the vocal cord), fracture of the cricoid cartilage, dislocation of an arytenoid cartilage, subglottic and glottic granulation tissue, and laryngotracheal stenosis (114). In some cases of difficult breathing it may be necessary to perform a tracheotomy (73, p. 208). This procedure does not necessarily result in permanent damage, but complications can occur especially in infants and young children (73, p. 208).

When a glottic web follows trauma, the glottis is shortened resulting in a high-pitched voice. In general, pitch is raised in direct proportion to the shortening of the free vocal cord margins (5).

Hoarseness, dysphonia, or aphonia may appear as a result of external laryngeal trauma. Direct trauma to the neck may occur in various sports activities such as baseball or in an automobile accident. In an automobile accident, injury to the neck often results from hitting the dash board or other obstructions within the car. Children are less apt to have external laryngeal and tracheal trauma in automobile accidents than adults (92). Trauma in children is more apt to be the result of normal play activities such as falling against a fence (92) or falling against the handle bars of a bicycle.

Voice therapy is recommended for various kinds of internal laryngeal trauma (59) and may be indicated after recovery from external trauma.

The Velopharyngeal Area, Oral Cavity, and Nose

Voice quality problems may be present in a child due to organic deviations in the velopharyngeal area, oral cavity, or nose. The presenting voice problem depends upon the physical site being misused. The most common problems are hypernasality and hyponasality.

The Velopharyngeal Area and Oral Cavity. The causes of velopharyngeal insufficiency include: (1) cleft palate, (2) short hard and/or soft palate, (3) an abnormally capacious pharynx, (4) partial or complete velar paralysis, and (5) submucous cleft palate. These causes can be present on congenital or developmental bases. The removal of tonsils and the adenoid many times reveals one or more of the last four conditions.

Velopharyngeal insufficiency may cause a voice problem characterized by combinations of hypernasality, hyponasality, and nasal emission (or snorting) of sounds. Sounds requiring a buildup of pressure within the mouth or pharynx are most frequently affected. Forty-three consonant sounds and blends are most frequently misarticulated because of velopharyngeal insufficiency (89) and are described in Chapter 3. The most common of the single consonants are /s/, /k/, /ʃ/, and /z/.

About 1 child in 750 live births has a cleft palate. Velopharyngeal insufficiency without an overt cleft palate ranges from 3.6% to 7.8% of the "cleft palate" population (47; 101; 104; 117). Cleft palates vary in extent of abnormality from a single cleft of the soft palate to bilateral clefts involving the soft and hard palate, the alveolar process, and the lip. After physical management many children need voice therapy to reduce hypernasality and nasal emission.

Various combinations of shortness of the hard and soft palate may occur. These are a short hard palate with a normal soft palate, a normal hard palate with a short soft palate, or a shortness of both the hard and soft palates (67). In some cases a child may have normal hard and soft palates but the pharyngeal area is abnormally deep making velopharyngeal closure impossible. Also structures may be normal in size and proportion, but a partial or complete paralysis may exist causing palate immobility, ineffective palate motion, or inconsistent palate motion (67).

Hypernasality is produced by relaxing the velum causing an opening into the nasopharyngeal port and using the nares as cul-de-sac resonators. Induced hypernasality is present when the velum is raised but is very tense and even thin. Here the velum acts as a drum head to increase nasality. A sluggish velum may cause assimilation nasality on sounds adjacent to the normally nasal sounds /m/, /n/, and /ŋ/.

Submucous cleft palate is a congenital deformity involving an imperfect muscle union across the velum (29). Arnold (4) described the characteristics of submucous cleft palate. He noted the uvula may be normal, or it may be bifid. The hard palate may have a triangular defect at its posterior border and this bony defect is covered by healthy looking mucosa which is very thin, however, because it is not supported by intervening musculature. Upon phonation the mucosal covering becomes stretched and the bony defect can be seen. Sometimes transilluminating the palate with a naso-pharyngoscope aids in the examination. The soft palate is usually too short and also weak so that it cannot elevate to produce nasopharyngeal closure.

A problem resembling cleft palate speech may occur after removal of the adenoid. Prior to the operation the velopharyngeal area functioned normally with the adenoid aiding in velopharyngeal closure. On the other hand, a child may have hyponasality immediately following removal of tonsils or adenoid because of postoperative edema. A waiting period of at least 3 weeks following the operation should be observed before attention to speech is given; by this time the edematous condition should be reduced and the hyponasality no longer present (113).

Wolski (136) discussed an adolescent girl with myasthenia gravis. The chief complaint was nasal emission and hypernasal speech. This condition was described as a neuromuscular transmission problem with an apparent blockage of nerve impulses from motor nerve endings across the synapse to the motor end plate of skeletal muscles. Hypernasality followed a specific pattern. The girl was quite free from symptoms in the morning but as the day progressed her voice became more and more nasal. Treatment for this condition was medical with various drugs being used to control nerve impulses.

It should be noted that many children with cleft palate have voice prob-lems in addition to hypernasality and nasal emission of air. The voice may sound hoarse and the laryngoscopic examinations often reveal the vocal cords to be hyperemic (reddened) and hyperplastic (thickened) (82).

Brooks and Shelton (25) found a greater percentage of cleft palate children with other voice problems than is usual for the general population. They found 10 % of 76 cleft palate children between the ages of 6 years 5 months and 12 years had voice defects other than or in addition to hyper-nasality, including breathiness, hoarseness, and inappropriate pitch level. On the other hand, Takagi, McGlone, and Millard (117) reported only 0.6 of 1 % of 1,061 patients (including 83 with non-cleft palatal insufficiency) had voice disorders other than hypernasality.

Bzoch (27) reported on 40 persons with cleft palate who received pha-ryngeal flap surgery. Before surgery, 14 of the subjects were judged to have breathy voice quality. Immediately following surgery this number dropped to 8 and by the end of the study only 2 cases appeared to have breathy voices. In the initial preoperative speech evaluation 7 of the 40 cases had hoarse voices. Laryngeal examinations revealed no lesions of the vocal cords. Following surgery 6 cases presented hoarse voices, which remained characteristic in 3 of the 7 cases at the time of final study. Breathiness in the voice is definitely reduced following such operative procedures, but hoarseness in the voice seems to persist in a certain number of such subjects.

Therefore, it would seem that attention by the speech clinician to hoarse quality in a cleft palate person is indicated.

McWilliams, Bluestone, and Musgrave (83) reported on laryngoscopic examinations of 32 children with cleft palate (19 boys and 4 girls, aged 4 years 10 months to 14 years 4 months) who had hoarse voices. Indirect laryngoscopy was done on 25 children with 7 children requiring direct laryngoscopy. Twenty boys and three girls had vocal nodules. Four other children had atypical laryngeal conditions including a posterior glottic chink, bilateral vocal cord hypertrophy, slight anterior edema, and improper approximation of the vocal cords.

The Nose. Hyponasality is a lack of proper nasal resonance. Arnold (4, p. 686) presented three cardinal diagnostic rules in assessing hyponasality: (a) the nasals /m/, /n/, and /ŋ/ always have a muffled sound, (b) nasal respiration, smell and taste are disturbed in the organic forms, and (c) disorders of swallowing do not occur. Hyponasality is usually due to an obstruction in the nasal or nasopharyngeal passages (39). Arnold (4, pp. 684–685) included among the causes deviated septum, bilateral turbinate hypertrophy, nasal polyps, enlarged adenoid tissue, allergic or inflammatory swelling of the mucosa, and traumatic injuries. He also stated hyponasal speech may be present on a functional basis, perhaps due to poor motor coordination, congenital dyspraxia, or faulty habits of verbal behavior. A hyponasal voice may persist long after the cause has been removed (122, p. 171).

In dealing with cases of hyponasality a thorough examination by the physician is essential. Surgical treatment is indicated when it is necessary to remove polyps or other obstructions causing the hyponasality. When swelling is present, congestion may be ameliorated by the use of medication (4, p. 686).

The Hearing Mechanism

Voice problems related to hearing loss vary considerably according to the type and degree of loss. In many cases the voice problem is so intertwined with problems of articulation and language it is difficult to describe the voice problem in isolation. These speech and voice problems are related to the child's imperfect and often distorted reception of the speech and voice of others and to difficulty in monitoring his own speech.

Problems related to the use of pitch have been described as typical of the person with a moderate or severe loss. Monotony of pitch is often mentioned (4, p. 637; 68, p. 412; 84; 100; 102, p. 297; 122) and a high fundamental pitch is frequent (4, p. 637; 17; 84; 112). Inappropriate loudness is due to difficulties in self-monitoring. There is a tendency for a person with a sensorineural loss to speak too loudly in order to hear his own voice, regardless of the background noise; a person with a conductive loss may speak too softly since his own voice reaches him by bone conduction and seems loud, while background noise seems soft to him (4, p. 637; 68, pp. 410–412; 102, pp. 296–297). Today, however, only a few children with conductive hearing losses and voice problems are seen by speech clinicians because of improved and more effective medical treatment for conductive hearing problems.

Resonance problems are common in the hearing impaired. A hollow, non-resonant quality has been mentioned (17; 52; 116). Hypernasality is often found in children with hearing losses (4, p. 637; 14, p. 283; 52, p. 100; 61; 100; 112; 116, p. 228). Hyponasal voices have been related particularly to conductive losses (4, p. 637; 97, p. 30).

Defective laryngeal tone, especially breathiness, is characteristic of hearing-impaired children (49; 60; 62; 100; 112; 116, p. 228). Children with hearing problems may have vocal nodules because of habitual misuse of the voice by strained speaking (4, p. 637) causing the voice to sound breathy or hoarse. Hearing-impaired children have slower than normal rate of speaking (17; 49; 61; 77; 119) and monotony in the rhythm of speech (4, p. 638; 52, p. 95; 61, p. 347).

Organic Changes Due to Vocal Abuse and Vocal Misuse

In the middle of the continuum of causation we have voice problems caused by vocal abuse and vocal misuse. Mismanagement of the laryngeal mechanism can cause damage to the vocal cords themselves and also can disturb the muscular coordination necessary for a good voice. Some vocal problems are directly caused by failure to inhibit the action of the extrinsic or swallowing muscles during the production of voice (137).

Either vocal abuse or vocal misuse may result in hyperfunction-hypofunction problems of voice. Brodnitz (21, p. 51) felt many voice disorders begin with excessive use of muscular force, which Froeschels (45) termed hyperfunction. After prolonged hyperfunctional use, the muscles become exhausted until they are unable to produce the normal degree of tonus and a weakening sets in (21, p. 51) and there is reduced adductor laryngeal action (6). Froeschels (45) called this stage hypofunction. von Leden (125) also stated persistent overexertion of the voice can cause weakness of the laryngeal muscles. Brodnitz (21, p. 51) pointed out hyperfunction usually involves the entire vocal mechanism although certain areas of the vocal mechanism may show more hyperfunction sites than others. Overexertion of the muscles of the larynx may cause irritation of the delicate tissues so they become swollen with blood (50, p. 197). Brodnitz (23) stated the excessive vocal strain used by a person who sings or speaks over a cold can set up a pattern of hyperfunctional voice usage that persists after the infection has disappeared; the pattern of excessive muscular exertion and excess breath pressure then becomes a habit. When hypofunction sets in after prolonged hyperfunction, the voice sounds breathy and the cords show a bowing indicating weakness of the thyroarytenoid muscles (21, p. 52).

Hyperfunctioning vocal practices may result in various pathological conditions in the larynx which cause the voice to sound hoarse, harsh, or breathy, or a combination of these features. These pathologies include vocal nodules, polyps, polypoid changes, vocal fold thickening, hyperkeratosis, nonspecific laryngitis, hematomas, hyperemia of the vocal cords, and hyperplasia of the vocal cords. If there are incorrect vocal practices plus infection, such as in chronic laryngitis, there may be changes in the larynx causing chronic inflammation known as chronic corditis (86, p. 671).

Incorrect use of the voice is called vocal abuse and vocal misuse. We separate them as two different abnormal vocal practices for etiological, evaluative, and voice therapy purposes. Vocal abuse (134) or poor vocal hygiene (31) includes traumatizing practices which may be quite detrimental. Vocal abuse is ". . . a combination of many injurious speech habits" (59). Common types of vocal abuse include shouting, screaming, cheering, strained vocalizations, excessive talking, reverse phonation, explosive release of vocalizations, abrupt glottal attack, throat clearing, coughing, and talking in the presence of high level noise. Cigarette smoking, intake of alcohol, and working in dusty places may also be considered vocally detrimental in some adolescents.

Vocal misuse refers specifically to improper use of pitch and loudness. Often there is an interplay between vocal abuse and vocal misuse with both present. Loud talking may accompany such vocal abuses as excessive talking and abrupt glottal attack. Vocal abuse and vocal misuse may be more pronounced in the living environment of some children. Loud talking families and large families are conducive to poor vocal habits. Many of the children Loré (79) studied with laryngeal dysfunction lived in an environment conducive to abuse and misuse of their voices.

Vocal Abuse

There are two types of vocal abuse, sudden and violent straining of the voice or continuous use of vocally abusive practices (69; 93). Froeschels (44) reported on a group of children under 16 years of age with various types of laryngeal dysfunction. There were 42 children with abrupt glottal attack, 15 children with too violent contraction of the pharyngeal constricting muscles, and 83 with both. Many undesirable vocal habits may originate in infancy and continue throughout childhood into adult life (137).

Some practices classified as vocal abuses have been subjected to study in the laboratory. Other vocal abuses have not been studied but clinical judgment tells us they are detrimental to the voice.

Let us look in detail at some of the vocal abuses.

Shouting, Screaming, Cheering. Shouting is extremely loud talking sometimes reaching 90 to 100 dB in intensity. A shout is "a loud burst of voice" (128, p. 804). In contrast to shouting, screaming means "to voice a sudden sharp loud cry . . . to produce harsh high tones . . ." which has ". . . a vivid startling effect" (128, p. 774) on listeners. Cheering is heard at sports events, on the playground, and in the gym. It is essentially ". . . a shout of applause or triumph" (128, p. 142). When a person screams, shouts, or engages in cheering excessive laryngeal tension is present which may result in irritation of the vocal cords. Shouting, screaming, and cheering are heard in children of all ages especially during play and during sports. A cheerleader may have voice problems, and many thousands of high school students are cheerleaders. Jensen (65) found 12 % of 377 female high school cheerleaders were judged to have hoarse voice quality. Shouting during sports activities is frequently heard in boys going through voice change (96, p. 8). Habits of screaming and shouting during play may cause chronic hoarseness (50, p. 198), disturbed muscular coordination necessary for phonation (46, p. 91), or vocal nodules (80, p. 158). Vigorous shouting and cheering may cause vascular engorgement, injury to muscles or laryngeal joints, or hematoma (86, p. 670). Children and adolescent boys are more likely to develop dysphonia than girls other than cheerleaders. This supports the general impression that boys tend to shout and cheer more strenuously than girls, probably due to the nature of their play and sports activities (53).

Brodnitz (21, p. 53) pointed out "sheer force is the main element in many voice disturbances. Children who use, and often misuse, their voices in youthful exuberance torture their vocal cords by shouting and yelling until screamers' nodules appear." The adolescent period is a time of muscular instability of the vocal mechanism when it should be free from all strain, yet it is the period when vocal exertion is likely to be very high; a youngster who returns from a ball game or other activity with huskiness, raspiness, and sometimes complete loss of phonation may be permanently damaging his voice (121).

Strained Vocalizations. Strained vocalizations include vocal imitation of cars, trucks, and airplanes during a child's play or when he is talking about noise sources. Usually extreme tension of the neck can be seen when strained vocalizations are made loudly. Strained vocalizations may produce hyperfunction in the vocal mechanism. This is evidenced by constriction of the muscles of the throat with the tongue sometimes thickened and pulled backward by contraction of its intrinsic muscles; in this instance the voice sounds restricted, strangulated, and harsh (21, p. 52).

Excessive Talking. A child who is vocally active doing much talking especially at a loud level and at an incorrect pitch is apt to have pathological changes in the larynx. West and Ansberry (130, p. 216) maintained that if the voice is properly used no amount of vigorous vocalization can damage the edges of the vocal cords. Rubin (107) stated with many singers "... vocal strain can occur from excessive use of even the most ideally produced voice ..." We maintain that prolonged vigorous talking by a child is a vocally abusive practice, sometimes resulting in vocal nodules (131). Further, talking with normal loudness and pitch excessively from morning to night is also a vocal abuse (93; 99, p. 866; 131; 132).

Reverse Phonation. Reverse phonation consists of vocalizing on the intake of air. It does not occur frequently during regular conversation or reading but usually during play and strenuous activities. Children typically do this as they play or imitate sounds of trains or trucks (134).

Explosive Release of Vocalizations. Explosive release of vocalizations occurs most often during play but is sometimes heard during quiet talking. It consists of building up air pressure in the subglottic area with the vocal cords tightly closed, followed by a sudden opening of the cords as a raucous vocalization is made. Many children build up excessive air pressure against the under surfaces of the vocal cords as they speak (130, p. 216) resulting in a staccato type of talking.

Abrupt Glottal Attack. The abupt glottal attack is referred to variously as the hard attack, harsh vocal attack, coup de glotte, glottal stroke, firm glottal attack, or glottal stop. It is the most commonly found faulty vocal production (37). The mechanical aspects of the abrupt glottal attack are essentially the same as an explosive release of vocalization. That is, in abrupt glottal attack there is a buildup of pressure and then a sudden release of the sound, but this is usually quite subtle compared to the loud expulsion of sound in an explosive type of release.

There are three different types of vocal attacks (80, p. 85; 96, p. 9): (1) the abrupt attack (including both the abrupt glottal attack and the explosive release), (2) the aspirate or breathy attack, and (3) the soft or normal attack. In the abrupt attack the vocal cords are firmly closed before the beginning of phonation, then subglottic air pressure is built up until there is a sudden release of the air pressure which produces a clicking noise. The trained ear can detect even the slightest degree of abrupt glottal attack (80, p. 85). In the aspirate or breathy attack the vocal cords are adducted to the paramedian line without a firm glottal closure. Thus there is escape of air accompanying the initiation of voice. In the soft or normal attack the vocal cords gradually begin to vibrate without any breathy sound or without the clicking noise of a sudden release. Clarity of tone depends upon the synchronous action of the expiratory and laryngeal muscles; this synchronous action results in a normal soft attack (39).

Types of glottal attack have been studied in the laboratory. Isshiki and von Leden (64) assessed air flow in the three types of vocal attack. There was no air flow observable before the onset of phonation in the abrupt glottal attack. In breathy or aspirate attacks, more than 150 cc of air were expelled before sound production began. In the normal soft attack between 30 and 100 cc of air were expelled before the actual start of phonation.

Koike, Hirano, and von Leden (71) studied 14 normal male adults as they phonated /ɑ/ for several seconds using abrupt, breathy, and soft initiation. Measurements were made as follows: "(1) Rise time of the pretracheal vibration . . . was defined to indicate the period from the onset of sound to the point at which the envelope amplitude reached the value of steady phonation. . . . (2) Air leakage before vocalization. (3) Time lag from the beginning of exhalation to the onset of sound. (4) Volume of air consumed during the initial 200 msec of phonation." Hard attack was associated with a short rise time and considerable air usage. The breathy vocal attack had the largest amount of air leakage prior to phonation compared to the other types of attack showing a definite time interval from beginning of air release to the initiation of phonation. Soft initiation was characterized by a long rise time and a small amount of air consumption.

Excessive use of the abrupt glottal attack results in irritation in the laryngeal area causing the voice to sound hoarse or harsh. Pathological changes, such as vocal nodules, may result from the overuse of this type of glottal attack. It may lead to hypofunctioning due to weakening of laryngeal muscles (21, p. 52). Koike and von Leden (72) studied vocal initiation in adults with laryngeal pathology and concluded ". . . 1) the abruptness of the initiation increases in pathological phonations, and 2) laryngeal tumors are especially related to abrupt initiation." They found the mean rise time for the tumor group was about the same as the abrupt initiation exhibited by normal laryngeal subjects; their unilateral paralysis group's rise time was approximately the same as breathy initiation in normal subjects. Thus we can assume that abrupt initiation is characteristic of those with various types of tumor including laryngeal papilloma and vocal cord polyps. This was a study of the laryngeal performance of adults with voice pathology which we are applying to children. However, we have found that children with vocal nodules characteristically use an abrupt glottal attack.

Coughing and Throat Clearing. Habitual, excessive, and hard coughing and vigorous and excessive throat clearing are common vocal abuses (46, p. 108; 96, p. 9; 133). Many children with laryngeal dysfunction have these vocal abuses. Senturia and Wilson (111) found a history of recurrent coughing in half of 92 school aged children with voice deviations. The percentage of children with a history of coughing was about the same for the group who had vocal cord lesions as for those who did not. Also vocal abuse may be associated with excessive laughing and crying. Analyses of high speed motion pictures of the larynx reveal vigorous changes in the larynx during even the mildest laughter or clearing of the throat (120). von Leden and Isshiki (126) studied laryngeal activities during coughing. An analysis of the high speed motion pictures indicated that a single cough impulse has three phases, ". . . an initial wide opening of the glottis, a protracted firm closure, and a complex vibratory (expiratory) phase." The vibratory or expiratory phase involves the vocal cords as well as the supraglottic structures and the mucosal lining of the posterior laryngeal wall. During a cough these structures undergo violent periodic undulations demonstrating the deleterious effect of a cough upon the delicate tissues of the larynx.

We have worked with children with vocal nodules who, with other vocal abuses, coughed excessively and vigorously. A cough may be a symptom of many different types of physical problems. An habitual hacking cough is symptomatic of allergic reactions to certain foods (85). An unusually long uvula sometimes causes a chronic cough, and it is sometimes amputated (34, p. 35). We knew a 7-year-old boy who had a persistent cough which the laryngologist felt was one of the vocal abuses contributing to the vocal nodule formation. An examination revealed a very long uvula hanging down into the pharynx and touching the base of the tongue The physician excised the tip of the uvula so it no longer caused a tickling irritation and the resulting cough. Schubert (110) also described this problem in two patients who had persistent coughs; the simple excision of part of the uvula under local anesthesia rid these patients of their coughs.

Frequent throat clearing is probably one of the most common vocal abuses. This may be due to a variety of medical problems, including allergy to ingested foods (85). Any possible medical reasons for this should be checked, but often it is present on an habitual basis.

Vocal Misuse (Pitch, Loudness)

The pitch and loudness of a child's voice need to be well controlled. Vocal misuse takes place when one or both of these aspects of voice is not used correctly. Usually we find children have habitual pitch and loudness levels within the range of acceptability. However, in some children traumatizing misuse occurs through the intermittent but frequent and daily use of too high and too loud voices. Of course, these misuses can be present in some children on a continual basis. These misuses may take place during talking and singing. Habitual excessive loudness is detrimental to the vocal mechanism. Isshiki, Okamura, and Morimoto (63) found distension of the trachea during loud phonation because of increased subglottal pressure. Thus we believe if excessive loud talking results in frequent distension of the trachea, muscle hyperfunctioning is created in this area. This can lead to chronic vocal abuse. The use of high intensity or high pitch levels when excited is indicative of general incorrect use of voice (99, p. 866). Vocal misuse may result in various types of laryngeal dysfunction characterized by harshness, breathiness, or hoarseness.

Talking in Noise. Both vocal abuse and vocal misuse occur when a person talks in the presence of noise. Vocal nodules are often found in workers who speak in high noise levels (36). The necessity for shouting to override excessive noise is enough to have a traumatic effect on the vocal cords if it continues over a period of time. However, the relationship of loudness and pitch is such that a person speaking in the presence of noise not only speaks loudly but also uses a higher pitch than he does habitually. Several studies have demonstrated an interrelationship between pitch and loudness.

What happens to loudness and pitch in a quiet environment? Brackett (18) measured pitch levels of young adults under four loudness levels, soft conversational, conversational, interphone-aircraft, and shouting. The average pitch levels rose a total of 82.4 Hz (10 semitones) from 119.4 Hz to 201.8 Hz. The rises from one level to another were 16.6 Hz (4 semitones), 18.8 Hz (2 semitones), and 47.0 Hz (4 semitones). Black (15), using 20 young adult males as subjects, had them say vowels and phrases. They were instructed to register 70, 80, 90, and 100 dB on a sound level meter; 70 dB was considered soft speech and 100 dB was considered loud speech. Rises in pitch with increased loudness were also measured in this study. The average total rise in pitch was 125 Hz (13 semitones) as the subjects went from 70 to 100 dB in loudness. The rise in pitch, however, was not equal among the different sound pressure levels studied. When the loudness increased from 70 to 80 dB there was a 13 Hz rise (2 semitones) in pitch, from 80 to 90 dB an additional 38 Hz rise (5 semitones), and from 90 to 100 dB an additional 74 Hz rise (6 semitones).

Ptacek and Sander (103), in their study of 80 young adults, asked subjects to take a deep breath and phonate the vowel /ɑ/ as long as possible while monitoring intensity on a volume unit (VU) meter with a microphone 2 inches from the mouth. Subjects were not asked to control the fundamental frequency of phonation. Soft phonation was held at 82 dB, moderate phonation 91 dB, and loud phonation 99 dB. The Hertz rises were as follows. For the men the three median frequency levels were soft phonation 120 Hz, moderate phonation up 14 Hz (1 semitone) to 134 Hz, loud phonation up 21 Hz (3 semitones) to 155 Hz, a total rise of 35 Hz (4 semitones). For the women the three median frequency levels were soft phonation 225 Hz, moderate phonation up 12 Hz to 237 Hz, loud phonation up 11 Hz to 248 Hz, a total rise of only 23 Hz (2 semitones).

Harris and Weiss (51) found in a group of adult male speakers there was an average increase in pitch of approximately 40 % for loud speech and a decrease in pitch of approximately 12 % for soft speech. Thus when we examine a child's use of pitch he should be observed when he is talking loudly, normally, and softly. When we decrease loudness we get a dividend in lowering the pitch level without paying much attention to the pitch itself.

We know high levels of noise are hazardous to hearing and should be avoided. We are especially interested in the misuse and abuse of the voice

TABLE 1

Effect of Noise on Voice Loudness and Pitch

Distance	Voice Loudness and Pitch			
	Normal Voice (70 dB) (Normal Pitch Level)	Raised Voice (80 dB) (Pitch Rises 13–17 Hz)	Very Loud Voice (90 dB) (Pitch Rises 14–38 Hz)	Shouting Voice (100 dB) (Pitch Rises 21–74 Hz)
	Noise Levels Which Interfere with Reception of Speech[a]			
feet				
½	71	77	83	89
1	65	71	77	83
2	59	65	71	77
3	55	61	67	73
4	53	59	65	71
5	51	57	63	69
6	49	55	61	67
12	43	49	55	61

[a] Speech interference levels (in decibels *re* 0.0002 dyne per cm²) which barely permit reliable conversation at the distances and voice loudness levels indicated.

when a person talks in a noisy environment. Talking in noise causes a person to talk louder as noise levels increase (48). We will present some of the studies done on noise in the environment in order to illustrate the effect environmental noise may have on the loudness, pitch level, and vocal abuse in the voice. We are interested especially in those situations where children and adolescents are apt to be talking for prolonged periods of time in high level noise. These situations include riding in automobiles, using farm machinery, and listening to rock music.

Shown in Table 1 is the effect of noise on loudness and pitch of the voice in adult males. The table is based on a report by Rosenblith *et al.* (106) which is based on reports by Beranek (12) and Beranek and Rudmose (13). The noise levels assume no reflecting surfaces nearby with the listener and talker facing each other. Two variables have been added to the table, voice intensity in decibels and Hertz rises in fundamental frequency as vocal intensity increases. The four loudness levels of voice shown are normal voice, raised voice, very loud voice, and shouting voice. The decibel levels for these speaking conditions are 70, 80, 90, and 100 dB (15). The Hertz rises between each intensity level are 13 to 17 Hz, 14 to 38 Hz, and 21 to 74 Hz (15; 18; 103). This table should be used conservatively because we have combined studies not originally designed to be combined. Also the use of the table is limited because the data is on adult males. Let's take an example of how this table might be used as a rough guide in an actual situation. If you are 3 feet away from a man talking in a normal voice at 70 dB, a noise level of 55 dB can be present before it begins to interfere with hearing his voice. If the noise level goes up to 61 dB it is necessary for him to raise the intensity of his voice to 80 dB with the fundamental frequency of his voice rising 13 to 17 Hz (2 to 4 semitones). As the noise increases to 67 dB it becomes necessary for him to talk at 90 dB while his fundamental frequency rises an additional 14 to 38 Hz (1 to 5 semitones). Then with the noise level at 73 dB a person has to talk at 100 dB and his voice rises an additional 21 to 74 Hz (3 to 6 semitones).

When riding in an automobile at high speeds it is necessary to talk in a very loud voice in order to be heard because of the level of noise created by the high speed movement of a car. The increase in loudness causes a rise in pitch, also an increased amount of vocal abuse. We have all had the experience of finding the volume of a car radio too loud when we slowed down from expressway speeds to 20 or 30 miles an hour on an exit ramp. Bolt, Beranek, and Newman, Inc. (16) measured the noise in automobiles. They found the amount of noise within automobiles went from 71 dB at 20 miles an hour to 78 dB at 40, and up to 82 dB at 60 miles an hour. According to our table, if the speaker is 1 foot from the listener, he would have to speak at a level of a shout at 100 dB to be heard when a car is traveling 60 miles an hour.

If the child with a voice problem lives in a farm community, the possibility of his talking in the presence of machine noise should be explored. Many young farm children ride for hours with their father on a tractor and at an early age begin to operate the tractor themselves often with another child riding with them. Talking in such conditions may have deleterious effects on the voice. Jones and Oser (66) found the noise level near the tractor operator's ear averaged 105 dB when the tractor was operated under full load. Ouzts (94) reported the noise level of three different pieces of farm machinery measured approximately 1 inch from the operator's ear on a plane parallel to the side of the head. Farm tractor noise was 96 dB sound pressure level (SPL), bean combine noise 102 dB SPL, and cotton picker noise 107 dB SPL. Also Lierle and Reger (76) found noise levels in farm tractors measured 6 inches from the ear ranged from approximately 85 dB SPL to 102 dB SPL (300 to 1200 Hz octave bands).

Talking while listening to rock bands may be detrimental to the voice. The intensity of rock bands has been measured and found to range from 85 dB SPL to 140 dB SPL with an average of 105 dB SPL to 110 dB SPL depending on the distance from a band (38; 78; 108). All the farm machinery and rock band levels are greater than the noise levels in Table 1 indicating a child talking in these noise conditions would have to use a shouting voice. The amount of talking in high level noise should be investigated when vocal abuse and vocal misuse are thought to be contributing to the cause of a voice disorder.

The Organic Changes

Vocal Nodules. The development of a vocal cord nodule usually involves three stages. First, a localized slight reddening appears on the free margin of the vocal cord with the submucosa showing dilation of the thin-walled blood vessels (135). This may be the sign of a very small hemorrhage (34, p. 126) or a mucous gland beginning to close (127). Second, there then occurs a localized swelling or thickening on the edge of the vocal cord (2; 74) with or without reddening. Third, a definite nodule forms with the thickening being replaced by fibrotic tissue and the nodule appears white, the same color as the free margin of the vocal cord (34, p. 126).

Sometimes inflammation is present around the area of the nodule. Figure 6 shows newly formed vocal nodules. They are concentrated and well defined and accompanied by a minimum of inflammation. Figures 7 and 8 show more mature nodules which are more diffuse with more inflammation present. The nodule ranges in diameter from one to several millimeters (135) with 3 mm being considered a very large vocal cord nodule. At no time is there any pain connected with this process from the very beginning to the formation of a mature fully formed vocal cord nodule (34, p. 126).

Vocal nodules may be unilateral or bilateral and are typically located on the edge of the free margin of the vocal cord in the area where there is

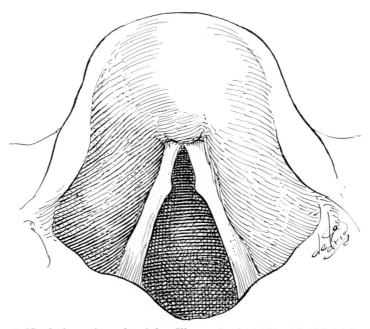

FIG. 6. Newly formed vocal nodules. Illustration by Melford D. Diedrick.

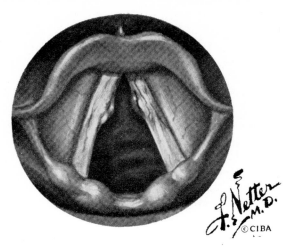

FIG. 7. Vocal nodules (inspiration). Copyright *Clinical Symposia* by Frank H Netter, M.D., published by CIBA Pharmaceutical Company.

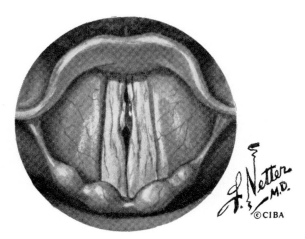

FIG. 8. Vocal nodules (phonation). Copyright *Clinical Symposia* by Frank H. Netter, M.D., published by CIBA Pharmaceutical Company.

maximum vibration, that is at the junction of the anterior and middle thirds of the vocal cord (21, p. 69; 125; 135). When vocal nodules are described as appearing in the middle third of the cord, this description does not include the nonvibrating or cartilaginous posterior third of the cord (the vocal process) (3; 5). Actually the nodules are at the same location in both descriptions. Often two nodules are exactly opposite each other and contact during phonation (34, p. 126). Size, composition, and location of the vocal nodules play an important part in the degree of hoarseness present. Extremely small nodules produce no symptoms, while others produce hoarseness (34, p. 126). Although a large mass generally produces more breathiness, a vocal nodule that is hard and not compressible can cause a faulty voice even though it is quite small (86, p. 662).

Each child with vocal nodules has to be studied thoroughly in order to establish the cause or causes so the proper treatment program can be outlined. Thus following the discovery of vocal nodules the question, "Why has this child developed this problem?" must be answered. The development of vocal nodules in children usually is the result of some sort of combination of (a) vocal abuse and vocal misuse, (b) chronic upper respiratory problems based on infections or allergies (2; 135), (c) the psychological living environment (home influence, size of family), (d) the physical living environment (air pollution), (e) the personality and general adjustment of the child (2; 135), and (f) endocrine imbalance especially thyroid (2; 135). Basic to all is a constitutional tendency toward development of vocal nodules (2; 69; 80, p. 176).

Vocal abuse and vocal misuse head the list of the basic reasons for the development of vocal nodules. They are ". . . visible organic changes that are the consequence of a functional disorder" (24). Specific misuse or abuse contributing to vocal nodules includes excessive laryngeal tension (96, p. 9), the habitual use of too high pitch (96, p. 8), the use of the voice at a pitch for which the larynx was not designed, as by cheerleaders and other speakers, prolonged vigorous use of the voice (86, p. 670), or simply the use of the voice for too many hours a day (135). Habitually using a loud voice seems to be responsible for vocal nodules in many cases with a history of talking in noise, talking to people with hearing losses or yelling at high levels of intensity (123, pp. 187–188). Long singing lessons (123, pp. 187–188), the use of improper methods of singing (93), and singing during acute inflammation of the cords contribute to the formation of vocal nodules (80, p. 178; 135).

Following is a case report of a child with vocal nodules (adapted from Wilson (131)). Billy was 5½ years old when his parents first noticed occasional hoarseness. During the next 6 months the periods of hoarseness became more and more frequent until the child continuously talked with a hoarse voice. Billy's pediatrician referred him to a laryngologist. The laryngeal examination revealed bilateral nodules about the size of a pinhead at the junction of the anterior and middle thirds of the vocal cords. A referral was made by the laryngologist to the speech clinic. During the initial interview the parents stated that Billy was an active boy liking sports and outdoor activities where much yelling, loud talking, and other forms of vocal abuse were noticed.

Voice analysis revealed that the child's conversational voice was hoarse in a mild to moderate degree. Under some conditions the voice sounded high in pitch and at times the voice was dysphonic and even aphonic especially at the ends of breath groups. Isolated vowels were analyzed for hoarseness. A psychological evaluation showed the child to be above average in intelligence with no evidence of emotional problems. Treatment was started with Billy on the basis of two sessions a week. The parents were counseled periodically about helping the child at home with carryover activities. After 3 months a laryngeal examination revealed a significant reduction in the size of the nodules. Treatment was continued for another 3 months when again the laryngologist reported a continuing reduction in the size of the nodules. During the next 6 months the sessions were gradually reduced in number from twice a week to once a month. A recheck by the laryngologist 1 year after treatment was started revealed the nodules had completely disappeared. The mother reported the child no longer had any undesirable vocal habits, his voice was free from hoarseness, and the pitch seemed generally lower. Periodic rechecks in the speech clinic during the following year indicated the child's voice was lower in pitch and completely free from hoarseness.

Polyps. Polyps of the vocal cord were described by Baker (9) as follows. They are the most common of the benign tumors of the larynx. They are not true tumors because they arise as the result of abuse of the larynx either from continued abuse or a single traumatic episode. A sudden violent use of the larynx can cause a submucosal hemorrhage and an organization of the hemorrhage into the formation of a tumor composed of connective tissue and blood. Degenerations lead further to a clearing of the blood with a formation of tissue liquid and a translucent appearance. The polyp increases in size with continued use of the voice. A polyp is usually single and is attached to the junction of the anterior and middle thirds of the vocal cord. It may be on top of the cord or on the edge of the cord. Sometimes the polyp is subglottic (Fig. 9) arising from the under edge of the vocal cord. The polyp may be one of two types, pedunculated or sessile (Figs. 10 and 11). Hoarseness varies according to the size and location of the polyp. The patient clears his throat frequently. The presence of a polyp requires increased effort in phonating and as a result the patient becomes exhausted when he does much talking.

Polypoid laryngitis, which according to Baker (9) is sometimes called chronic hypertrophic laryngitis and polyposis of the vocal cords, results from the continued misuse and abuse of the voice. He stated that this is a condition in which small vocal nodules undergo degeneration into small polypoid tumors which eventually involve the entire edge and the surface of both cords (Fig. 12). This condition is more common in adults than children.

Dysphonia Plicae Ventricularis. In some cases severe voice alteration

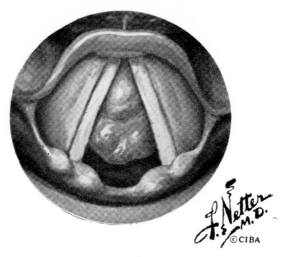

FIG. 9. Subglottic polyp. Copyright *Clinical Symposia* by Frank H. Netter, M.D., published by CIBA Pharmaceutical Company.

is due to dysphonia plicae ventricularis which is the use of the false vocal cords instead of the true vocal cords for phonation. It is also called ventricular phonation and hyperkinesia of false cords (Fig. 13). As DeWeese and Saunders (34, p. 110) stated this condition is a common cause of hoarseness frequently overlooked. The voice symptoms are quite distinct in this type of problem with the voice usually lower than normal in pitch with a restricted pitch range and with some characteristics of vocal fry present. Usually the laugh, the cry, and the cough are unaffected. Laryngeal examination reveals according to Fred (42) that during quiet breathing the false cords appear normal although often thickened. When a person is asked to phonate, the false vocal cords close and are seen to vibrate. This problem may be due to vocal abuse, vocal misuse, or psychological stress; it may follow an operation; it may be present on a congenital basis with true vocal cords present or on a congenital basis in the absence of true vocal cords.

Vocal abuse and misuse can result in such severe pathology of the true vocal cords that a person is forced to use the false vocal cords for phonation. Talking in this manner may be temporary until the pathology of the true vocal cords is resolved or the person may continue to use ventricular phonation on an habitual basis. In psychogenic ventricular dysphonia the false cords are used for phonation even though the true vocal cords themselves are intact. This may occur according to Brodnitz (21, p. 77) after severe attacks of laryngitis or after removal of benign tumors of the true vocal cords. Thus the patient sometimes without being aware of it is afraid to use his vocal cords and substitutes ventricular phonation for true vocal

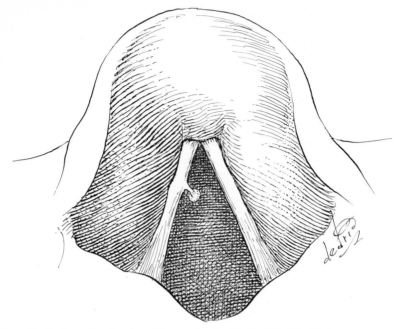

Fɪɢ. 10. Pedunculated polyp. Illustration by Melford D. Diedrick.

cord phonation; this causes the person to tire easily and to complain about pains while speaking (21, p. 77). Insecurity or neurosis may be the cause of this type of ventricular cord phonation (43).

Ventricular phonation may follow operations. Parisier and Henneford (95) reported on an 11-year-old boy who had had three operations for the removal of juvenile laryngeal papillomas, one operation at 4 years of age and two at 5 years of age. After the last two operations the child developed persistent hoarseness and mild dyspnea on extreme exertion. At 11 years of age a laryngeal web was discovered and removed. When his voice showed only minimal improvement during the next 6 months the laryngologist noted the child phonated with the false vocal cords and voice therapy was recommended for development of a more adequate voice. Obviously the elimination of false vocal cord phonation was the goal of voice therapy.

Hyperkeratosis. The beginning hyperkeratotic lesion in adults according to Cracovaner (32) is a small red thickening on the edge of a vocal cord. It may be either on the anterior third or middle third of the vocal cord or both (Fig. 14). He felt hyperkeratotic lesions are due to chronic irritation including overindulgence in alcohol, excessive smoking, abuse of the voice, and inhalation of dust and fumes. Laryngeal examinations of elementary school children in the Baynes and Wendling (11) study revealed hyper-

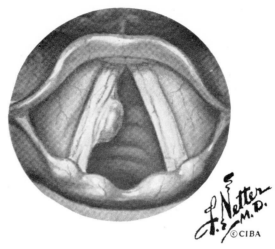

Fig. 11. Sessile polyp. Copyright *Clinical Symposia* by Frank H. Netter, M.D., published by CIBA Pharmaceutical Company.

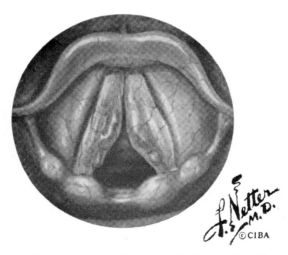

Fig. 12. Polypoid degeneration of true cords. Copyright *Clinical Symposia* by Frank H. Netter, M.D., published by CIBA Pharmaceutical Company.

keratotic plaques on the edges of the vocal cords in 57 of 242 children with harsh or breathy voices. Hyperkeratotic lesions in children are no doubt due to abuse of the voice, inhalation of dust and fumes, or chronic infection of the sinuses or pharynx. Baynes and Wendling (11) described a hyperkeratotic plaque as a somewhat irregular white thickening of the mucosa, on the edge of the middle third of the vocal cord with the cord showing evi-

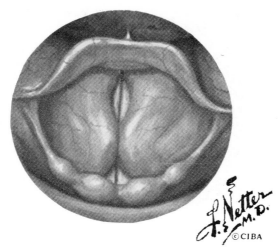

FIG. 13. Hyperkinesia of false cords. Copyright *Clinical Symposia* by Frank H. Netter, M.D., published by CIBA Pharmaceutical Company.

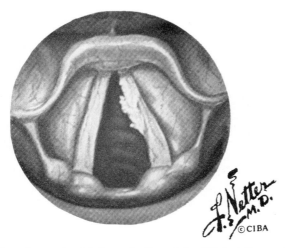

FIG. 14. Hyperkeratosis of left cord. Copyright *Clinical Symposia* by Frank H. Netter, M.D., published by CIBA Pharmaceutical Company.

dence of inflammation. Rosedale and Nowara (105) described hyperkeratosis as a "... typical pearly raised thickening of the mucosa with apparently normal movement of the vocal cords."

Nonspecific Laryngitis. In nonspecific or chronic laryngitis there is thickening and reddening of the vocal cords due to vocal abuse (Fig. 15). The diagnosis of nonspecific laryngitis can be made if vocal abuse can be

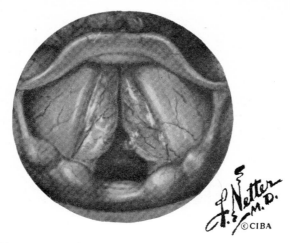

Fig. 15. Edematous vocal cords in chronic laryngitis. Copyright *Clinical Symposia* by Frank H. Netter, M.D., published by CIBA Pharmaceutical Company.

demonstrated and all possible sources of infection or irritation excluded (21, p. 68). Hoarseness is a primary symptom. There may be no indicated medical treatment with voice therapy proving beneficial when vocal abuse and vocal misuse are the factors maintaining the nonspecific laryngitis (124).

Contributing Causes

A variety of conditions may be contributing causes to voice problems present on a functional basis, an organic basis, or on the basis of organic conditions resulting from vocal misuse and abuse. These contributing conditions include glandular conditions, allergies, upper respiratory conditions (chronic pharyngitis, sinusitis, deviated nasal septum), prepubertal and pubertal disturbances, and premenstrual tension. These contributing causes are intertwined with the three basic causes of voice problems, in fact it may be difficult to find the exact relationship of causes. For example, an allergic tendency is a common symptom in childhood vocal nodules (46, p. 107). The following case history illustrates this.

A 10-year-old boy had been periodically hoarse for the past 5 years. The indirect laryngeal examination revealed essentially normal laryngeal structures except for nonspecific laryngitis with the vocal cords red and swollen. Further exploration revealed two reasons for the laryngitis: allergy to airborne pollens (present most of the year where he lived) and excessive shouting and loud talking when playing. Antihistamines were prescribed to relieve the edematous condition of the vocal cords. Voice therapy was administered by a speech clinician for the purposes of reducing vocal abuse during play, eliminating the use of abnormally high pitch, and teaching the boy to use correct loudness in all situations. Within a period of 6 months the combination of medical and voice therapy resulted in a voice much improved in quality with the periodic hoarseness eliminated (134).

Glandular Conditions

Metabolic disorders due to a dysfunction of the endocrine glands should be carefully investigated because the endocrine condition may affect laryngeal structures. For example, an enlargement of the larynx may be seen in certain malfunctions of the anterior pituitary gland (26). Also hoarseness or huskiness may be present in myxedema and thyroid and parathyroid tumors (26). A chronically high-pitched voice in a male is usually functional but may be caused by the larynx failing to develop to a normal size because of glandular difficulties, for example hypogonadism (86, p. 658). Vocal quality may be influenced by changes in metabolic and hormonal balances (20) with a low metabolic rate resulting in a retention of body fluids in the surface tissues in the laryngeal and tracheal areas (19).

Allergy

Allergic sensitivity to both airborne and ingested substances may contribute to voice problems through swelling of the mucosa of the nose, mouth, throat, larynx, trachea, and lung structures. In some of these areas there also may be hyperemia, a reddening due to increased blood concentration. Reactions to allergic symptoms may include such vocal abuses as chronic coughing and throat clearing which in turn aggravate the swelling and inflammation and may result in organic changes. The swelling and reddening of the mucosa of the nose may result in hyponasality (4, p. 684). Brodnitz (19) estimated that at least 3 % of the population in the United States has some form of respiratory allergy which may influence laryngeal function. Senturia and Wilson (111) found a family history of allergy present in about 25 % of the children with laryngeal dysfunction.

Respiratory allergy may result from airborne irritants such as pollens (134), dust (41; 87, p. 99), powdered substances of various kinds (87, p. 99), and chemical substances (41). Ingested allergens include foods and liquids. The mucous membrane lining of the mouth, throat, and larynx are likely to be the primary shock organs of ingested substances (85). In some cases the contact may be relatively brief but when it is repeated frequently, drinking milk for example, allergic reactions may result (85). The lingering coating effect on the mucosa of some dairy products, especially high fat milk and ice cream, results in increased time for allergic reaction to take place. Milk and ice cream of low fat content are preferable as they have little coating effect. Because food remains in the body for hours antigens can be absorbed from the intestinal tract reaching the mucosa through the circulatory system thus causing a delayed allergic reaction (85). Consultation with an allergist is indicated when allergy is suspected.

Upper Respiratory Conditions

Infections of the upper respiratory tract are a source of laryngeal difficulties (32; 125). In the presence of impaired nasal respiration and the resulting mouth breathing, the mucous covering of the cords becomes dry leaving the cords unprotected (69). Purulent postnasal discharge bathing the vocal cords has often been observed in patients with vocal nodules (69). Sinusitis is often an accompanying problem in cases of chronic laryngitis (91). Kelly and Craik (69) found marked nasal obstruction or sepsis in 23 % of their cases with vocal nodules. Senturia and Wilson (111) noted in their studies of voice deviant children about one-half of the children had increased amounts of mucus, pus, or mucopus in each nasal fossa.

Prepubertal and Pubertal Changes in the Voice

During puberty there is normally a change in the habitual pitch level of the voice due to growth changes in the larynx. This process is called mutation. Most children, both boys and girls, go through voice change without any residual voice problems. However, in some instances there is disturbed mutation. Luchsinger (80, p. 193) classified disturbed mutation in boys according to three clinical forms: (1) delayed mutation—the vocal changes do not take place until several years later than usual; (2) prolonged mutation—a persistence of the clinical signs of voice change over several years instead of just a few months; (3) incomplete mutation—the voice does not fully develop into the normal voice of an adult. In all three forms the voice is characterized by high pitch, chronic hoarseness, and many voice breaks. Since the normal change in a girl's voice is a lowering of only 3 or 4 semitones her voice may not be considered deviant if it does not change although she may be considered to have a rather high-pitched and childish voice. However, if the pitch of her voice lowers significantly a pitch problem develops called perverse mutation. A mutational bass voice may occur in a preadolescent boy who has forced his voice down even lower than normal through imitating adults with very low pitches (129). A boy over 14 or 15 years of age with a high-pitched voice is usually classified as being effeminate. It is possible to confuse the use of effeminate pitch inflections after the voice has changed with the problem of persistent falsetto. Therefore, before attempting to lower pitch the speech clinician should make sure the older male teenager really has a too high habitual pitch not just effeminate sounding pitch inflections.

Many voice problems arise during the period of voice change. Harrington (50, pp. 192–193) stated, "Many of the voice disorders of the adult have their origin in the period of adolescence and are outgrowths of the voice problems related to this rather crucial period." Brodnitz (21, p. 56) noted many deviations of voice found in the adult can be traced back to voice change during puberty.

Causes of Disturbed Mutation

Mutational disturbances of the voice are based on organic or functional causes or a combination of both. Organic bases include laryngeal asymmetries (129), small vocal cords (39), congenital or acquired anterior laryngeal web which shortens the cords (5), incomplete mutation in girls complaining of irregular menstruation (80, p. 194), and endocrine disturbances (39; 80, p. 188; 129). However, ordinary laryngoscopy usually reveals no major abnormalities in cases of suspected endocrine pathology (80, p. 188). Functional causes of disturbed mutation include psychological involvements (5; 120), sexual conflict related to a protest against social or sexual maturity (122, p. 165), and infantile or juvenile personality (5; 80, p. 196; 122, p. 160). A high-pitched voice may be used as a defense against pitch breaks or as a method of preventing a hoarse voice (122, p. 166). The physical examination usually shows normal sexual development in mutational falsetto voices (5; 80, p. 195).

Laryngeal Findings. In functional mutational disturbances the laryngological examinations are negative as far as size, structure, and function of the larynx are concerned. Hyperemia or congestion of the vocal cords may be present (3; 5; 80, p. 196), but these signs are the result not the cause of the habitual use of the falsetto voice (80, p. 196). Allen and Peterson (1) presented a case report of an 18-year-old male with a falsetto voice who had considerable inflammation of the entire laryngeal area. After pitch had been lowered to a normal level this inflammation was greatly relieved. They felt that in this case the inflammation had been caused by his use of a falsetto voice.

In mutational disturbances the glottis assumes a typical oval shape upon phonation and in some instances the posterior half of the glottis may close incompletely (5). The mechanical reason for mutational falsetto voice is the functional overcontraction of the cricothyroid muscles; as a result there is a pronounced elevation of the entire larynx during phonation (5).

Singing during Mutation. In general both boys and girls should be discouraged from choral singing during mutation (21, p. 60; 80, p. 159; 129). This is particularly true for boys who show voice breaks (21, p. 60). Brodnitz (21, p. 60) stated as a rule the singing voice requires a year or two longer to develop than the speaking voice. He advised that formal singing training should not be started in boys before the age of 17 or 18 and in girls not before 16 years of age. Overexertion of the intrinsic muscles of the larynx while singing may cause permanent impairment of the vocal coordination necessary in phonation (46, p. 91). The untrained singer may develop laryngeal symptoms which may be temporary or permanent if he persists in singing in outdoor classes, at summer camp, in the church choir, and in other situations for which he is not trained (8). Rubin (107) mentioned the following as conditions likely to result from abusive singing: acute laryngitis because of infection or trauma to the vocal cords, chronic vocal corditis, vocal nodules, circumscribed or diffuse submucosal hemorrhage, and hypofunction or myasthenia resulting from deterioration in the tonus of the laryngeal muscles. We have worked with several adolescents who had misused their voices during singing and developed hypofunction manifesting itself in a bowing of the vocal cords during phonation.

Premenstrual Tension

Hoarseness may be associated with premenstrual tension. Edematous conditions occurring a few days preceding the menstrual period may cause an increase in the bulk of the vocal cords and result in lowered pitch and vocal instability with voice breaks (40). This hoarseness or vocal instability occurring for a few days each month should not be of concern to the speech clinician. Therefore, if hoarseness is noted in surveying girls who have started menstruation, a recheck should be made at some other time during the month and inquiry made about the periodicity of the hoarseness.

Functional Causes

In a functional voice disorder there is nothing wrong with the vocal mechanism. Even though a child has a healthy larynx, oral structures, and a healthy body the use of pitch, loudness, or voice quality is inadequate. The voice problem for example may be present on a psychological basis or may be the result of imitation. Many children with voice abnormalities have no visible dysfunction or pathology upon laryngoscopy. This problem according to Moore, White, and von Leden (88) may be due to unusual or abnormal vibratory patterns of the vocal cords in the absence of actual pathology. A functional voice disorder may be characterized by normal laryngoscopic examination results with or without abnormal stroboscopic examination results; the dysphonia is more severe than any lesions or inflammations appear to warrant; and the problem may be of nervous origin but may in turn be conducive to the formation of organic lesions (98). A functional voice disorder is reversible and disappears when the vocal organs are used correctly (98). Functional causes of voice problems of children can be divided into three categories, (1) psychological factors, (2) imitation, and (3) faulty learning.

Psychological Factors

Functional voice disorders, especially those of deviations in flexibility, quality, pitch, and loudness, may be explained as a result of psychological disturbance or maladjustment (33, p. 208). We have discussed functional mutation problems. Psychological factors which may cause a functional voice disorder in children include personality differences, character defects, emotional disturbances, and disturbed parent-child relationships. These factors are overlapping and intertwining and are not always easily separated. At times we see children with voice problems quite directly related to only one of the factors, but in many children a disturbance is seen in more than one factor. Murphy (90, p. 32) discussed disturbed parent-child relationships as a cause of voice problems. He stated, "Many of the apprehensions or anxieties connected with vocal dysfunctions are traceable to disturbed earlier child-adult relationships, at least in part." He felt positive identification between parent and child is necessary to establish efficient communication between them and if this identification malfunctions and the parent has an undesirable voice quality, he becomes a negative model, with the child developing ". . . anxiety-reducing behavior, some of which may take the form of psychogenic voice symptoms."

Psychological factors may result in a variety of vocal symptoms. Some of these are hoarseness, harshness, breathiness, hypernasality, loudness problems, aphonia, and hypertense voice problems. For example, over-aggressiveness may be one of the personality differences resulting in an habitually too loud voice (102, p. 112). Hoarseness can be closely related to emotional disturbances or psychic trauma (125). A child who is unmanageable and hyperactive may have a rough hoarse voice reflecting a character defect, congenital or acquired. When a child is emotionally disturbed, either neurotic or psychotic, almost any type of voice problem may be present.

Aphonia is a loss of voice which is usually present on a psychosomatic basis (75; 81; 125) and is commonly referred to as hysterical aphonia. The lack of voice may be the presenting symptom of a major emotional disturbance with aphonia representing an avenue of escape from a difficult dilemma (81). Hysterical aphonia in children before the age of adolescence is very rare, but dysphonia in the absence of vocal strain is relatively common in children and may be considered an hysterical symptom (46, p. 147). Barton (10) described the syndrome of hysterical dysphonia. The condition may vary from a mild dysphonia to complete loss of voice. He described a distinct clinical type called *whispering dysphonia* which is most commonly found in women and may appear any time between puberty and menopause. The patient speaks in a halting whisper without hoarseness and at times the phonation is normal. Most of Barton's case descriptions are of adult patients although he refers to one girl 16 years of age. During the laryngeal examination, according to Barton, the vocal folds move properly, they approximate accurately, and are free from any tumors or inflammations.

Excessive laryngeal tension may be caused by emotional conflicts (96, p. 9). Any type of personality conflict may be revealed in a hyperfunctional voice problem. Some children have bowed vocal cords as the result of an hysterical condition. In some patients with deviant voice patterns including complete aphonia a mirror examination of the vocal cords shows a bowing and imperfect approximation in phonatory effort typical of hypofunctioning resulting from hyperfunctioning; this appears even though the midline approximation usually occurs in coughing or laughing (75).

Various psychological factors or upsets may be a factor in vocal abuse and vocal misuse. The result may be the formation of vocal nodules. Heaver (53) obtained psychiatric evaluations of 50 patients ranging in age from $3\frac{1}{2}$ to 73 years. The vocal cords of each of these patients were reddened, swollen, and thickened or had nodules or polyps with hyperkinetic action of the vocal cords. He concluded disordered emotional states tend to engender vocal abuse which could result in nodules or edematous fibromata. Callahan (28) also said many people who exhibit abuse of the vocal cords have emotional strain and insecurity in their immediate background. He presented a report of an investigation of 20 adults with varying degrees of abuse of the vocal cords who had not been able to develop a normal voice after operation for benign tumor. The results of psychological projective tests revealed unstable emotional reactions including inadequacy, anxiety, and hostility. Callahan concluded continued vocal abuse is caused by emotional disturbances characterized by unconscious conflicts and frustrations.

Imitation

Murphy (90, pp. 31–32) contended, "Throughout the vocal learning process, the voice acquired by the child depends upon how he imitates or identifies with important adults in his environment." He further stated the amount of pleasure a child gets from his early vocal play will influence how well he can master normal vocalization. He pointed out for normal growth preverbal language including babbling and vocal play must receive approval and success early in the child's life.

It is possible for a child to have a voice problem as a result of imitation of others with voice problems in his environment (102, p. 112). Klinger (70), for example, wrote about a child who imitated a cousin's cleft palate speech. Van Riper (122, p. 167) stated stereotyped inflections may be due to foreign language influence.

Faulty Learning

An overly loud voice is not necessarily a sign of overaggressiveness but sometimes a result of poor speech habits (35). The patient may have no organic lesion to account for the inefficient vocal cord vibration causing breathy voice (35). Murphy (90, p. 33) cited as an example of faulty learning the child who has parents with hearing losses and who may be required to raise loudness and pitch levels and thus develop a pitch or quality disorder.

We have seen the causes of voice problems exist in many dimensions. The causes of a specific voice problem are intertwined among the organic and functional with vocal abuse and vocal misuse strongly associated factors. Plans for examinations and therapy are based on the constellation of causes present in a child. We will proceed with examinations in the next chapter.

REFERENCES

1. Allen, B., and Peterson, G. E. Laryngeal inflammation in a case of falsetto. *J. Speech Dis.*, **7**, 1942, 175–178.
2. Arnold, G. E. Vocal nodules. In J. F. Daly (Moderator), Voice problems and laryngeal pathology. *New York J. Med.*, **63**, 1963, 3096–3110.
3. Arnold, G. E. Clinical application of recent advances in laryngeal physiology. *Ann. Otol.*, **73**, 1964, 426–442.
4. Arnold, G. E. Physiology and pathology of speech and language. In R. Luchsinger and G. E. Arnold, *Voice-speech-language. Clinical communicology: Its physiology and pathology.* Belmont: Wadsworth Publishing Company, 1965.
5. Arnold, G. E. Advances in laryngeal physiology and their clinical application. *Eye, Ear, Nose, Throat Monthly*, **45**, 1966, 78–84.
6. Aronson, A. E., Peterson, H. W., Jr., and Litin, E. M. Voice symptomatology in functional dysphonia and aphonia. *J. Speech Hearing Dis.*, **29**, 1964, 367–380.
7. Baker, D. C., Jr. Congenital disorders of the larynx. *New York J. Med.*, **54**, 1954, 2458–2462.
8. Baker, D. C., Jr. Laryngeal problems in singers. *Laryngoscope*, **72**, 1962, 902–908.
9. Baker, D. C., Jr. Polypoid vocal cord. In J. F. Daly (Moderator), Voice problems and laryngeal pathology. *New York J. Med.*, **63**, 1963, 3096–3110.
10. Barton, R. T. The whispering syndrome of hysterical dysphonia. *Ann. Otol.*, **69**, 1960, 156–164.
11. Baynes, R. A., and Wendling, D. Clinical observations of children with voice disorders. *Asha*, **7**, 1965, 393.
12. Beranek, L. L. Airplane quieting. II. Specification of acceptable noise levels. *Trans. Amer. Soc. Mech. Engin.*, **69**, 1947, 97–100.
13. Beranek, L. L., and Rudmose, H. W. Sound control in airplanes. *J. Acoust. Soc. Amer.*, **19**, 1947, 357–364.
14. Berg, F. S. Educational audiology. In F. S. Berg and S. G. Fletcher (Editors), *The hard of hearing child.* New York: Grune and Stratton, 1970.
15. Black, J. W. Relationships among fundamental frequency, vocal sound pressure, and rate of speaking. *Lang. Speech*, **4**, 1961, 196–199.
16. Bolt, Beranek, and Newman, Inc. Noise in automobiles: Report on a second set of tests conducted by Bolt, Beranek, and Newman, Inc. for J. Walter Thompson Company and the Ford Motor Company on 29 April 1965. Report No. 1249, Job No. 181176, 14 May 1965.
17. Boone, D. R. Modification of the voices of deaf children. *Volta Rev.*, **68**, 1966, 686–792.
18. Brackett, I. P. Intelligibility related to pitch. *Speech Monogr.*, **13**, 1946, 24–31.
19. Brodnitz, F. S. Voice problems of the actor and singer. *J. Speech Hearing Dis.*, **19**, 1954, 322–326.
20. Brodnitz, F. S. The holistic study of the voice. *Quart. J. Speech*, **48**, 1962, 280–284.
21. Brodnitz, F. S. *Vocal rehabilitation.* Ed. 3. Rochester, Minn.: American Academy of Ophthalmology and Otolaryngology, 1965.
22. Brodnitz, F. S. Review of A. T. Murphy, *Functional voice disorders. J. Commun. Dis.*, **1**, 1967, 100–101.

23. Brodnitz, F. S. Semantics of the voice. *J. Speech Hearing Dis.*, **32**, 1967, 325–330.
24. Brodnitz, F. S., and Froeschels, E. Treatment of vocal nodules by chewing method. *Arch. Otolaryg. (Chicago)*, **59**, 1954, 560–565.
25. Brooks, A. R., and Shelton, R. L., Jr. Incidence of voice disorders other than nasality in cleft palate children. *Cleft Palate Bull.*, **13**, 1963, 63–64.
26. Burke, H. A., Jr. Endocrine aspects of otolaryngology. *Laryngoscope*, **78**, 1968, 857–862.
27. Bzoch, K. R. The effects of a specific pharyngeal flap operation upon the speech of forty cleft-palate persons. *J. Speech Hearing Dis.*, **29**, 1964, 111–120.
28. Callahan, N. Vocal cord strain. *Southern Med. J.*, **51**, 1958, 1578–1584.
29. Calnan, J. Submucous cleft palate. *Brit. J. Plast. Surg.*, **6**, 1954, 264–282.
30. Cavanagh, F. Vocal palsies in children. *J. Laryng.*, **69**, 1955, 399–418.
31. Cooper, M., and Nahum, A. M. Vocal rehabilitation for contact ulcer of the larynx. *Arch. Otolaryg. (Chicago)*, **85**, 1967, 41–46.
32. Cracovaner, A. J. Hyperkeratosis of the larynx. *Arch. Otolaryg. (Chicago)*, **70**, 1959, 287–291.
33. Curtis, J. F. Disorders of voice. In W. Johnson and D. Moeller (Editors), *Speech handicapped school children*. Ed. 3. New York: Harper and Row, 1967.
34. DeWeese, D. D., and Saunders, W. H. *Textbook of otolaryngology*. Ed. 3. St. Louis: C. V. Mosby Company, 1968.
35. Fabricant, N. D. Some facts about dysphonia. *Eye, Ear, Nose, Throat Monthly*, **41**, 1962, 729–738.
36. Ferguson, G. B. Organic lesions of the larynx produced by misuse of the voice. *Laryngoscope*, **65**, 1955, 327–336.
37. Flower, R. M. Voice training in the management of dysphonia. *Laryngoscope*, **69**, 1959, 940–946.
38. Flugrath, J. M. Modern-day rock-and-roll music and damage-risk criteria. *J. Acoust. Soc. Amer.*, **45**, 1969, 704–711.
39. Fomon, S., Bell, J. W., Lubart, J., Schattner, A., and Syracuse, V. R. Otolaryngology and speech therapy. *Eye, Ear, Nose, Throat Monthly*, **45**, 1966, 71–76.
40. Frable, M. A. S. Hoarseness, a symptom of premenstrual tension. *Arch. Otolaryg. (Chicago)*, **75**, 1962, 66–68.
41. Frank, D. I. Hoarseness: New classification and brief report of four interesting cases. *Laryngoscope*, **50**, 1940, 472–478.
42. Fred, H. L. Hoarseness due to phonation by the false vocal cords: Dysphonia plicae ventricularis. *Arch. Intern. Med. (Chicago)*, **110**, 1962, 472–475.
43. Freud, E. D. Functions and dysfunctions of the ventricular folds. *J. Speech Hearing Dis.*, **27**, 1962, 334–340.
44. Froeschels, E. Laws in the appearance and the development of voice hyperfunctions. *J. Speech Dis.*, **5**, 1940, 1–4.
45. Froeschels, E. Hygiene of the voice. *Arch. Otolaryg. (Chicago)*, **38**, 1943, 122–130.
46. Greene, M. C. L. *The voice and its disorders*. Ed. 2. Philadelphia: J. B. Lippincott Company, 1964.
47. Gylling, U., and Soivio, A. I. Submucous cleft palates. Surgical treatment and results. *Acta Chir. Scand.*, **129**, 1965, 282–287.
48. Hanley, T. D., and Steer, M. D. Effect of level of distracting noise upon speaking rate, duration and intensity. *J. Speech Hearing Dis.*, **14**, 1949, 363–368.
49. Hardy, W. G., Pauls, M. D., and Haskins, H. L. An analysis of language development in children with impaired hearing. *Acta Otolaryg. (Stockholm)*, *Suppl. 141*, 1958.
50. Harrington, R. Children with voice disorders. In W. Johnson (Editor), *Speech problems of children*. New York: Grune and Stratton, 1950.
51. Harris, C. M., and Weiss, M. R. Effects of speaking condition on pitch. *J. Acoust. Soc. Amer.*, **36**, 1964, 933–936.
52. Haycock, G. S. *The teaching of speech*. Stoke-on-Trent, England: Hill and Ainsworth, Ltd., 1933. Reprintings by Volta Bureau, Washington, D. C.

53. Heaver, L. Psychiatric observations on the personality structure of patients with habitual dysphonia. *Logos*, **1**, 1958, 21–26.
54. Holinger, P. H., and Brown, W. T. Congenital webs, cysts, laryngoceles and other anomalies of the larynx. *Ann. Otol.*, **76**, 1967, 744–752.
55. Holinger, P. H., Johnston, K. C., Conner, G. H., Conner, B. R., and Holper, J. Studies of papilloma of the larynx. *Ann. Otol.*, **71**, 1962, 443–447.
56. Holinger, P. H., Johnston, K. C., and Kodros, A. C. Vocal cord paralysis in infants. *Eye, Ear, Nose, Throat Monthly*, **40**, 1961, 109–113.
57. Holinger, P. H., Johnston, K. C., and McMahon, R. J. Hoarseness in infants and children. *Eye, Ear, Nose, Throat Monthly*, **31**, 1952, 247–251.
58. Holinger, P. H., Johnston, K. C., and Schiller, F. Congenital anomalies of the larynx. *Ann. Otol.*, **63**, 1954, 581–606.
59. Holinger, P. H., Schild, J. A., and Maurizi, D. G. Internal and external trauma to the larynx. *Laryngoscope*, **78**, 1968, 944–954.
60. Hudgins, C. V. Voice production and breath control in the speech of the deaf. *Amer. Ann. Deaf*, **82**, 1937, 338–363.
61. Hudgins, C. V., and Numbers, F. C. An investigation of the intelligibility of the speech of the deaf. *Genet. Psychol. Monogr.*, **25**, 1942, 289–392.
62. Irwin, R. B. Education of the hard of hearing child in Ohio. *Hear. News*, **17**, 1949, 5–7.
63. Isshiki, N., Okamura, H., and Morimoto, M. Maximum phonation time and air flow rate during phonation: Simple clinical tests for vocal function. *Ann. Otol.*, **76**, 1967, 998–1007.
64. Isshiki, N., and von Leden, H. Hoarseness: Aerodynamic studies. *Arch. Otolaryng. (Chicago)*, **80**, 1964, 206–213.
65. Jensen, P. J. Hoarseness in cheerleaders. *Asha*, **6**, 1964, 406.
66. Jones, H. H., and Oser, J. L. Farm equipment noise exposure levels. *Amer. Industr. Hyg. Ass. J.*, **29**, 1968, 146–151.
67. Kaplan, E. N., Jobe, R. P., and Chase, R. A. Flexibility in surgical planning for velopharyngeal incompetence. *Cleft Palate J.*, **6**, 1969, 166–174.
68. Keaster, J. Impaired hearing. In W. Johnson and D. Moeller (Editors), *Speech handicapped school children*. Ed. 3. New York: Harper and Row, 1967.
69. Kelly, H. D. B., and Craik, J. E. Laryngeal nodes and the so-called amyloid tumour of the cords. *J. Laryng.*, **66**, 1952, 339–358.
70. Klinger, H. Imitated English cleft palate speech in a normal Spanish speaking child. *J. Speech Hearing Dis.*, **27**, 1962, 379–381.
71. Koike, Y., Hirano, M., and von Leden, H. Vocal initiation: Acoustic and aerodynamic investigations of normal subjects. *Folia Phoniat. (Basel)*, **19**, 1967, 173–182.
72. Koike, Y., and von Leden, H. Pathologic vocal initiation. *Ann. Otol.*, **78**, 1969, 138–147.
73. Laupus, W. E., and Pastore, P. N. The larynx. In E. L. Kendig, Jr. (Editor), *Disorders of the respiratory tract in children*. Philadelphia: W. B. Saunders Company, 1967.
74. Levbarg, J. J. Vocal therapy versus surgery for the eradication of singers' and speakers' nodules. *Eye, Ear, Nose, Throat Monthly*, **18**, 1939, 81–82, 91.
75. Lewy, R. B. Practical aspects of psychiatry applied to otolaryngology. *Arch. Otolaryng. (Chicago)*, **77**, 1963, 444–446.
76. Lierle, D., and Reger, S. The effect of tractor noise on auditory sensitivity of tractor operators. *Ann. Otol.*, **67**, 1958, 372–388.
77. Linder, G. Uber den zeitlichen verlauf der sprechweise be gehorlosen. *Folia Phoniat. (Basel)*, **14**, 1962, 67–76. Cited by S. P. Quigley. Language research in countries other than the United States. *Volta Rev.*, **68**, 1966, 68–83.
78. Lipscomb, D. M. High intensity sounds in the recreational environment: A hazard to young ears. *Clin. Pediat. (Phila.)*, **8**, 1969, 63–68.
79. Loré, J. M., Jr. Hoarseness in children. *Arch. Otolaryng. (Chicago)*, **51**, 1950, 814–825.

80. Luchsinger, R. Physiology and pathology of respiration and phonation. In R. Luchsinger and G. E. Arnold, *Voice-speech-language. Clinical communicology: Its physiology and pathology.* Belmont: Wadsworth Publishing Company, 1965.
81. McCaskey, C. H. Aphonia. *Ann. Otol.,* **55,** 1946, 524–530.
82. McDonald, E. T., and Baker, H. K. Cleft palate speech: An integration of research and clinical observation. *J. Speech Hearing Dis.,* **16,** 1951, 9–20.
83. McWilliams, B. J., Bluestone, C. D., and Musgrave, R. D. Diagnostic implications of vocal cord nodules in children with cleft palate. *Laryngoscope,* **79,** 1969, 2072–2080.
84. Martony, J. On the correction of the voice pitch level for severely hard of hearing subjects. *Amer. Ann. Deaf,* **113,** 1968, 195–202.
85. Missal, S. C. Food allergy in the ear, nose and throat practice of allergy. *Laryngoscope,* **51,** 1961, 512–523.
86. Moore, G. P. Voice disorders associated with organic abnormalities. In L. E. Travis (Editor), *Handbook of speech pathology.* New York: Appleton-Century-Crofts, Inc., 1957.
87. Moore, G. P. *Organic voice disorders.* Englewood Cliffs: Prentice-Hall, Inc., 1971.
88. Moore, G. P., White, F. D., and von Leden, H. Ultra high speed photography in laryngeal physiology. *J. Speech Hearing Dis.,* **27,** 1962, 165–171.
89. Morris, H. L., Spriestersbach, D. C., and Darley, F. L. An articulation test for assessing competency of velopharyngeal closure. *J. Speech Hearing Res.,* **4,** 1961, 48–55.
90. Murphy, A. T. *Functional voice disorders.* Englewood Cliffs: Prentice-Hall, Inc., 1964.
91. Murphy, R. S. Hoarseness. *Nova Scotia Med. Bull.,* **46,** 1967, 177–179.
92. Novick, W. H. Traumatic stenosis of the trachea in children. *Laryngoscope,* **57,** 1967, 1351–1357.
93. Orton, H. B. The significance of hoarseness. *New Orleans Med. Surg. J.,* **103,** 1951, 511–515.
94. Ouzts, J. W. Auditory temporary threshold shift following exposure to high-intensity and variable-peaked farm machinery noise. *J. Auditory Res.,* **9,** 1969 64–70.
95. Parisier, S. C., and Henneford, G. E. Surgical correction of acquired vocal cord webs. *Arch. Otolaryng. (Chicago),* **90,** 1969, 103–107.
96. Peacher, G. Voice therapy for ulcers and nodules of the larynx. In *Proceedings of the first institute on voice pathology, and the first international meeting of laryngectomized persons.* Cleveland Hearing and Speech Center, 1952.
97. Penn, J. P. Voice and speech patterns of the hard of hearing. *Acta Otolaryng. (Stockholm), Suppl. 124,* 1955.
98. Perello, J. Dysphonies fonctionnelles: Phonoponose et phononevrose. *Folia Phoniat. (Basel),* **14,** 1962, 150–205. Cited by A. E. Aronson, H. W. Peterson, Jr., and E. M. Litin. Voice symptomatology in functional dysphonia and aphonia. *J. Speech Hearing Dis.,* **29,** 1964, 367–380.
99. Perkins, W. H. The challenge of functional disorders of voice. In L. E. Travis (Editor), *Handbook of speech pathology.* New York: Appleton-Century-Crofts, Inc., 1957.
100. Peterson, G. E. Influence of voice quality. *Volta Rev.,* **48,** 1946, 640–641.
101. Porterfield, H. W., and Trabue, J. C. Submucous cleft palate. *J. Plast. Reconstr. Surg.,* **35,** 1965, 45–50.
102. Pronovost, W., and Kingman, L. *The teaching of speaking and listening in the elementary school.* New York: Longmans, Green and Company, 1959.
103. Ptacek, P. H., and Sander, E. K. Maximum duration of phonation. *J. Speech Hearing Dis.,* **28,** 1963, 171–182.
104. Rees, T. D., Wood-Smith, D., Swinyard, C. A., and Converse, J. M. Electromyographic evaluation of submucous cleft palate: A possible aid to operative planning. *J. Plast. Reconstr. Surg.,* **40,** 1967, 592–594.

105. Rosedale, R. S., and Nowara, R. J. Etiology of hoarseness with an original classification. *Ohio Med. J.*, **56**, 1960, 334–338.
106. Rosenblith, W. A., Stevens, K. N., and the staff of Bolt, Beranek, and Newman, Inc., *Handbook of acoustic noise control. Vol. II. Noise and man*, Wright Air Development Center Technical Report 52-204, 1953.
107. Rubin, H. J. Role of the laryngologist in management of dysfunctions of the singing voice. *Trans. Pacif. Coast Otoophthal. Soc.*, **45**, 1964, 57–77.
108. Rupp, R. R., and Koch, L. J. Effects of too-loud-music on human ears—But, Mother, rock'n roll HAS to be loud! *Clin. Pediat. (Phila.)*, **8**, 1969, 60–62.
109. Saunders, W. H. The larynx. *Clin. Sympos.*, **16**, 1964, 67–99.
110. Schubert, K. Cough due to a large uvula. *German Med. Monthly*, **8**, 1963, 413.
111. Senturia, B. H., and Wilson, F. B. Otorhinolaryngic findings in children with voice deviations. *Ann. Otol.*, **77**, 1968, 1027–1041.
112. Silversmith, R. S. Articulation and voice analyses of preschool hard of hearing children. Unpublished master's project, State University of New York at Buffalo, 1970.
113. Sloan, R. F., Brummett, S. W., Westover, J. L., Ricketts, R. M., and Ashley, F. L. Recent cinefluorographic advances in palatopharyngeal roentgenography. *Amer. J. Roentgen.*, **90**, 1964, 977–985.
114. Smith, R. O., Hemenway, W. G., English, G. M., Black, F. O., and Swan, H. Post-intubation subglottic granulation tissue: Review of the problem and evaluation of radiotherapy. *Laryngoscope*, **79**, 1969, 1227–1251.
115. Sokoloff, M., and Rieber, R. W. Phonatory and resonatory problems. In R. W. Rieber and R. S. Brubacker (Editors), *Speech pathology. An international study of the science*. Philadelphia: J. B. Lippincott Company, 1966.
116. Streng, A., Fitch, W. J., Hedgecock, L. D., Phillips, J. W., and Carrell, J. A. *Hearing therapy for children*. Ed. 2. New York: Grune and Stratton, 1958.
117. Takagi, Y., McGlone, R. E., and Millard, R. T. A survey of the speech disorders of individuals with clefts. *Cleft Palate J.*, **2**, 1965, 28–31.
118. Tarneaud, J. The fundamental principles of vocal cultivation and therapeutics of the voice. *Logos*, **1**, 1958, 7–10.
119. Tato, J. M., and Arcella, A. I. La inteligibilidad en funcion della velocidad de la palabra hablada en los sordos desmutizados. *Acta Otorinolaring. Iber. Amer.*, **23**, 1962, 551–560. Cited by S. P. Quigley. Language research in countries other than the United States. *Volta Rev.*, **68**, 1966, 68–83.
120. Timcke, R., von Leden, H., and Moore, P. Laryngeal vibrations: Measurements of the glottic wave. Part II. Physiologic variations. *Arch. Otolaryng. (Chicago)*, **69**, 1959, 438–444.
121. Uris, D. Teen talk. *Todays Speech*, **10**, 1962, 15–16.
122. Van Riper, C. *Speech correction. Principles and methods*. Ed. 4. Englewood Cliffs: Prentice-Hall, Inc., 1963.
123. Van Riper, C., and Irwin, J. V. *Voice and articulation*. Englewood Cliffs: Prentice-Hall, Inc., 1958.
124. Van Thal, J. H. Dysphonia. *Speech Path. Ther.*, **4**, 1961, 11–21.
125. von Leden, H. The clinical significance of hoarseness and related voice disorders. *J. Lancet*, **78**, 1958, 50–53.
126. von Leden, H., and Isshiki, N. An analysis of cough at the level of the larynx. *Arch. Otolaryng. (Chicago)*, **81**, 1965, 616–625.
127. Voorhees, I. W. The nonsurgical treatment of aphonia (hoarseness). *New York J. Med.*, **34**, 1934, 53–55.
128. *Webster's seventh new collegiate dictionary*. Springfield, Mass.: G. C. Merriam, 1963.
129. Weiss, D. A. The pubertal change of the human voice. *Folia Phoniat. (Basel)*, **2**, 1950, 127–158.
130. West, R. W., and Ansberry, M. *The rehabilitation of speech*. Ed. 4. New York: Harper and Row, 1968.

131. Wilson, D. K. Children with vocal nodules. *J. Speech Hearing Dis.*, **26**, 1961, 19–26.
132. Wilson, D. K. Voice re-education of children with vocal nodules. *Laryngoscope*, **72**, 1962, 45–53.
133. Wilson, D. K. Voice re-education in benign laryngeal pathology. *Eye, Ear, Nose, Throat Monthly*, **45**, 1966, 76–80.
134. Wilson, D. K. Voice therapy for children with laryngeal dysfunction. *Southern Med. J.*, **61**, 1968, 956–958.
135. Withers, B. T. Vocal nodules. *Eye, Ear, Nose, Throat Monthly*, **40**, 1961, 35–38.
136. Wolski, W. Hypernasality as the presenting symptom of myasthenia gravis. *J. Speech Hearing Dis.*, **32**, 1967, 36–38.
137. Zerffi, W. A. C. Functional vocal disabilities. *Laryngoscope*, **49**, 1939, 1143–1147.

3

EXAMINATIONS

Children with voice problems require special examinations. The findings form the basis upon which voice therapy is planned. Many specialists may be involved. The most effective procedure for examining children with voice disorders is in the framework of a team situation.

The Voice Team

Examinations of children with voice problems include those made by various specialists in a team situation. A team approach assures comprehensive care of children with voice problems from the time the problems are first discovered through examination, consultation, treatment, and follow-up. Before a voice therapy program begins it is necessary to coordinate the relevant examinations conducted by the team. For example, a child with a chronically hoarse voice will require a head and neck examination. He may also need a general physical examination, an audiological evaluation, and examinations and tests for allergy. The child may need psychiatric or psychological attention, the parents may need counseling, and the child may need voice therapy.

We advocate a team approach to the diagnosis and treatment of children with voice problems to coordinate these services in an efficient and effective manner. Every major center of population should have a voice team similar to a cleft palate team, and a hearing team described by Wilson (112).

Support for the team approach to diagnosis and treatment of voice disorders comes from many sources. Moore (66) emphasized the need of a child with a voice problem for an overall approach. O'Neill and McGee (74) felt a team approach should be used. Brodnitz (18, p. 78) emphasized the necessity for close cooperation between the speech clinician and the laryngologist. He stated (18, p. 80) vocal rehabilitation requires a total approach and emphasis should be placed on the medical, functional, and psychological factors present in a person with a vocal disturbance.

Baynes (6) and Freeman (35; 36) described the team approach in the public schools of Oakland County, Michigan. One aspect of this service is especially for children who have chronic voice disorders. Four or five times a year the consulting laryngologist examines children for abnormalities of the vocal cords. Local speech clinicians attend these examinations to review findings and to formulate recommendations with the examining physician. Their team includes the otolaryngologist, the teachers, parents, principals, psychologists, school social workers, and school nurses.

Organization of Voice Team

A team approach to children with voice problems may be organized in different ways. It may function successfully with as few as two continuing members, a laryngologist and a speech clinician, with arrangements for referral or consultation with other specialists as circumstances dictate. We feel, however, the ideal voice team is one in which specific members of the team meet regularly scheduling half-day sessions as frequently as the number of children with serious voice deviations warrants. The specialties represented at any one team meeting depend on the problems of the children being seen. This type of team approach is advocated with the realization that a more loosely knit organization may be adequate in some communities.

A team coordinator schedules and plans the sessions. Typically the coordinator is either a laryngologist or a speech clinician. The team coordinator establishes a roster of all specialists who might be called upon to examine, diagnose, and treat children with voice problems and to conduct follow-up examinations as necessary. In addition to the speech clinician and laryngologist other specialists who may serve as members or consultants to the team include a pediatrician, neurologist, psychiatrist, psychologist, audiologist, social worker, and school personnel. Children are referred to the team by any of its members or by other specialists. The team approach includes four stages: initial evaluation, team staffing, progress evaluations, and follow-up. At a single meeting the team members may see children in any stage.

Stage I: Initial Evaluation. A list of children with voice problems is accumulated by the coordinator. The coordinator and one other team member, the laryngologist and the speech clinician, meet on a regular basis. At these meetings they select the tests and examinations indicated for each child. The coordinator informs the parents of the recommended tests and examinations and it is the parents' responsibility to see that the child is examined by the specialists of their choice. For example, the following may be recommended: a head and neck examination, a voice examination, a general physical examination, and psychological evaluations. Any immediate treatment indicated is given as the child is seen by each specialist. For example, a child may need medication to relieve allergic conditions affecting the nose and throat.

Stage II: Team Staffing. After the examinations have been completed the coordinator accumulates all the reports. The team members actively concerned with the group of children under consideration then meet for a staffing. The children are presented at this time with some team members demonstrating the results of their detailed examinations. As the members of the team look over his shoulder the laryngologist can show them the child's vocal nodules. The speech clinician may wish to conduct a brief session with the child to demonstrate the child's vocal capabilities and disabilities. Each member of the team presents his report. The team then decides on the overall treatment for the child. The parents are informed of the planned course of action, and when indicated and appropriate the child is told of the treatment plan.

Stage III: Progress Evaluations. All children are scheduled at regular intervals in the course of their treatment for team evaluation and impressions of their progress. These evaluations include rechecking pathologies and evaluating effectiveness of certain therapies. Some children are seen by the team when a team member runs into specific problems requiring discussion and decisions by the team. Questions may arise about certain aspects of the treatment and other team members may make suggestions for a change in treatment. Decisions about dismissal from active treatment are also made by the team.

Stage IV: Follow-up. Following formal or regular aspects of treatment the child is seen periodically by the team. Usually children are rechecked every 3 to 6 months. The number of rechecks depends upon the problem and the child. This follow-up assures carryover of new voice habits and freedom from physical or psychological complaints. Following is a case illustration of the four team stages (adapted from Wilson (114)).

An extremely active and loud-talking 6-year-old boy was first seen by a school speech clinician during a kindergarten speech and voice survey. His voice was hoarse especially after periods of excessive loud talking and shouting during games. The school speech clinician consulted with the coordinator of the local voice team who was a speech clinician in the city speech and hearing center. They met with a laryngologist and the following recommendations were made: general physical examination, head and neck examination, neurological examination, and voice tests (Stage I).

Results of these examinations were presented at a team staffing (Stage II) as follows. A laryngeal examination revealed small nodules on the free margin of each vocal cord at the junction of the anterior one-third and posterior two-thirds. The laryngologist felt these vocal nodules were due to improper use of the voice and were too small for removal. The general physical and neurological examinations were negative. The voice tests revealed the child had a moderate to severe hoarseness, a too high habitual pitch, an excessively loud voice, and many vocal abuses including shouting, screaming, strained vocalizations when imitating jet planes and racing cars, and explosive release of vocalizations. The physicians prescribed a mild tranquilizer to help the child relax. The social worker agreed to see the parents for counseling in an effort to help the child reduce his excessive activity. The psychologist reported the child was essentially emotionally stable and of normal intelligence. Voice therapy was recommended and the speech clinician saw the child for 16 voice therapy sessions of 45 min each over a period of 3 months. Vocal abuse and loud talking were given attention and his habitual pitch level was lowered. During this period the child was seen by the team after 10 voice therapy sessions for a progress evaluation (Stage III) at the request of the speech clinician and laryngologist. The purpose was to demonstrate improvement in the boy's voice and show that the nodules were definitely reduced in size. He was also seen after the 16 sessions for another progress evaluation at which time he was dismissed from active voice therapy. The period of intensive voice therapy was followed by a series of check-ups to insure continuation of improved speaking habits (Stage IV). A laryngeal examination 6 months after the initiation of voice therapy revealed the vocal nodules were reduced in size. Another laryngeal examination a year later showed they were no longer present.

The voice team is the most desirable approach to the rehabilitation of children with voice problems. The comprehensive team approach can be adapted to the needs of a specific community.

Head and Neck Examination

The head and neck examination includes a careful evaluation of the neck, ears, nose, oral cavity, nasopharynx, and larynx. Special attention is given to those areas related to the chief complaint connected with the voice problem.

Neck

According to Saunders (87, p. 80) palpation of the neck is part of the complete examination of the larynx and is described as follows. A cyst of the thyroglossal duct may be felt by the physician in the space between the thyroid cartilage and the hyoid bone. The space between the thyroid and cricoid cartilages is palpated to check for lymph nodes; the space is shortened as the patient prolongs /i/ at a high pitch showing normal function of the cricothyroid muscle and its nerve supply, the superior laryngeal nerve. The neck is palpated for swelling and enlargement of lymph nodes which may reveal glandular disease. The sternocleidomastoid muscles are checked for lymph nodes. The shape of the thyroid cartilage is noted (29, p 21).

Ears

The ears are carefully examined using the following procedures described by Collins (25, pp. 83–86). The physician first examines the external ear noting inflammatory spots, fissures, or ulcers. The back of the ear is examined especially for eczema. The ear canal is next examined, the physician pulls the ear upward, outward, and backward and inserts an aural speculum. The ear canal is inspected. Inflammations, discharges, and amount of wax are noted. The tympanic membrane is carefully inspected. It should be slightly concave and pearly grey with a lustrous surface. Normally the handle of the malleus can be seen near the center of the membrane. The short process of the malleus can be seen in the upper third of the membrane. In a retracted membrane the handle of the malleus appears foreshortened and the short process prominent (25, p. 322). Any perforations of the membrane are noted (25, p. 88). Fluid in the middle ear can be seen if the membrane is fairly transparent (25, p. 89).

Nose

Collins (25, pp. 76–79) described the physician's examination of the nose. A nasal speculum is inserted into a nostril and the naris spread for better viewing. The septum is examined. It should be smooth and pink located centrally in the nose and not deviated to one side. The turbinates are examined for swelling. Nasal polyps and mucopus are noted. If the mucous membrane of the nose is purplish and boggy, especially with excess mucoid secretion, an allergic condition is suspected.

Oral Cavity

DeWeese and Saunders (29, pp. 11–13) described the physician's examination of the mouth. The tongue is inspected and palpated. It should be red and not coated. The frenum is checked for length and is normal if the patient can protude the tongue between the teeth. The floor of the mouth is examined and palpated for growths. The salivary glands are examined for normalcy. The teeth are checked for cavities and abscesses and gingivae for freedom from bleeding. The palatine or faucial tonsils should not project beyond the tonsillar pillars. The posterior pharyngeal wall is examined by depressing the tongue with a tongue depressor. Examination of this area includes noting the amount of mesial movement in the lateral pharyngeal walls during phonation (95). The size of the nasopharyngeal isthmus is noted (22).

The hard and soft palates are carefully examined. They should show a distinct difference in color, the soft palate pink and the hard palate whiter; the uvula can be bifid (29, pp. 13–14). The relationship in length of the hard and soft palates is evaluated. Arnold (3, p. 662) pointed out the soft palate is normally about half as long as the hard palate; however, in cases of congenital velar insufficiency it may be only a third or a fourth as long. The hard palate may be disproportionately shortened in varying degrees in the presence of a normal soft palate (50). In some cases, both the hard and soft palates may be short. The soft palate is carefully inspected for movement. This includes checking the symmetry of movement during the eleva-

tion of the soft palate and noting whether there is general or localized movement during phonation (95). The physician palpates the palate to detect
absence of muscle union in the soft palate and a notch in the hard palate
which may indicate a submucous cleft of the palate (22). Calnan (22) noted
that intraoral examination of a submucous cleft palate reveals a short
palate and a large nasopharyngeal isthmus. The uvula is often bifid or gives
the impression it is bifid because it may look more broad and squat than
usual with a "gutter" running down it. There is also a definite "gutter"
along the midline of the velum with the median raphe absent. Further the
velum fails to occlude the nasopharyngeal isthmus, but its mobility and
degree of elevation are not markedly impaired although the velum may not
elevate during swallowing as it does in a person with a normal palate.
Calnan (22) stated a submucous cleft palate should not be confused with
other types of palatal insufficiencies such as congenital short palate. He
pointed out the median raphe of the velum is usually well marked in the
congenital short palate indicating a sound muscle union, although nasality
is usually present since the nasopharyngeal isthmus appears to be large and
the velum may elevate inadequately and asymmetrically.

Intranasal transillumination aids in the diagnosis of submucous cleft
palate. During this procedure the midline defect of muscle union is seen as
a bright area which extends anteriorly to a notch in the hard palate (22).
Massengill (60) described a special technique for doing this. A light source
is placed in a nostril and a photoelectric cell is placed under the palate. Light
is registered on the photoelectric cell if a submucous cleft is present.

Calnan (22) listed another type of velopharyngeal insufficiency described
as cerebral agenesis which results in hypernasality and poor speech. In these
cases the palate moves poorly or not at all. There is no history of neural
disease or evidence of other paralysis although Calnan noted there is sometimes a weakness of the muscles of the lips and tongue. If this condition is
suspected, the examiner can have the patient sustain vowels such as /ɑ/
while the examiner notes whether the velum continues to be in an upward
position throughout the sustained phonation; a muscle weakness may be
indicated if the velum relaxes during sustained phonation (12).

Nasopharynx

DeWeese and Saunders (29, pp. 15–16) described the examination of the
nasopharynx. A postnasal mirror is inserted into the pharynx almost
touching the posterior pharyngeal wall. The examiner views the posterior
opening of the nose and the posterior end of the vomer located centrally in
the opening. The turbinates are viewed. Drainage from the maxillary sinus
may be seen. The adenoid (pharyngeal tonsil) grows from the roof and
posterior wall of the nasopharynx. Increased size of the adenoid may
occlude the eustachian tubes and obstruct nasal breathing.

Subtelny and Koepp-Baker (98) stated the peak of lymphatic growth of the adenoid is somewhere between 9 or 10 years of age and 14 or 15 years of age. The adenoid can first be seen in x-rays at about 6 months to 1 year becoming quite well defined at 2 years. By adulthood adenoid atrophy is usually complete. This normal atrophy is gradual and slow and when all structures otherwise are normal the palate and the pharyngeal wall can make increasingly compensatory movements in order to maintain adequate velopharyngeal closure (98). After adenoidectomy during childhood there usually is a brief period of 2 or 3 weeks of hypernasal speech. Occasionally hypernasality persists when some patients are left with a capacious nasopharynx or when a submucous cleft palate is unmasked.

Larynx

Indirect Laryngoscopy. Indirect or mirror laryngoscopy requires a laryngeal mirror, a head mirror with a good light source, 2-×2-inch gauze, and an alcohol lamp (57, p. 386). The patient is asked to sit in an erect position with the base of the spine snugly against the back of an examining chair (57, p. 386). The knees should be held together and the chin slightly forward (29, p. 17). The patient is asked to relax his shoulders, neck, and arms and to breathe regularly and moderately deeply to minimize gag reflex and throat spasm (57, p. 386). A laryngeal mirror, No. 3 to No. 6 depending on oropharyngeal width, is warmed over an alcohol lamp and its temperature tested on the back of the physician's hand. The patient protrudes his tongue; the examiner using a piece of gauze gently grasps the tongue between the thumb and middle finger; the index finger is used to retract the upper lip (57, p. 386). As the laryngeal mirror is inserted into the pharynx the uvula and soft palate are pressed upward (29, p. 18). Emphasis is placed on having the patient breathe quietly through the mouth, if necessary panting like a dog will help prevent gagging (29, p. 18). The physician examines the larynx during breathing and during phonation of a prolonged high-pitched /i/ (29, p. 18). Loré (57, p. 388) suggested the following check list in examining the larynx: (1) vocal cords (free edges and superior surfaces) and their motion, (2) arytenoid cartilages and their motion, (3) ventricles and ventricular bands, (4) anterior and posterior commissures, (5) subglottic space (wall of trachea), (6) aryepiglottic folds, (7) lingual and laryngeal surfaces and free edges of epiglottis, and (8) the glossoepiglottic folds. Structural deviations, motion problems, and pathology are carefully noted and described.

Figure 16 shows the high points of the laryngeal examination. For more detailed explanation of the head and neck examination the reader is referred to Loré (57), DeWeese and Saunders (29), and Collins (25).

Direct Laryngoscopy. Young children who cannot be examined by indirect laryngoscopy because of lack of cooperation or an extreme gag

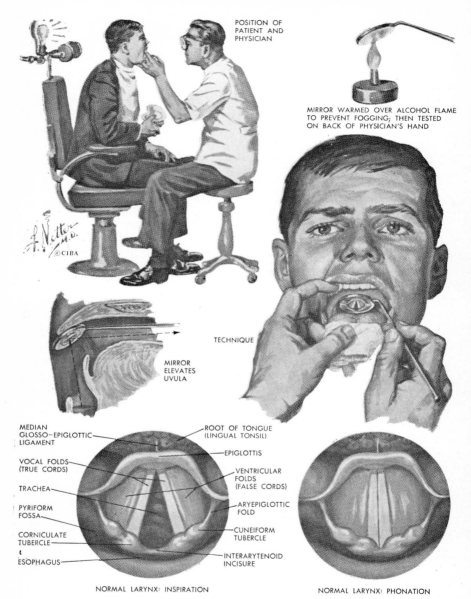

POSITION OF
PATIENT AND
PHYSICIAN

MIRROR WARMED OVER ALCOHOL FLAME
TO PREVENT FOGGING; THEN TESTED
ON BACK OF PHYSICIAN'S HAND

TECHNIQUE

MIRROR
ELEVATES
UVULA

MEDIAN
GLOSSO-EPIGLOTTIC
LIGAMENT

VOCAL FOLDS
(TRUE CORDS)

TRACHEA

PYRIFORM
FOSSA

CORNICULATE
TUBERCLE

ESOPHAGUS

ROOT OF TONGUE
(LINGUAL TONSIL)

EPIGLOTTIS

VENTRICULAR
FOLDS
(FALSE CORDS)

ARYEPIGLOTTIC
FOLD

CUNEIFORM
TUBERCLE

INTERARYTENOID
INCISURE

NORMAL LARYNX: INSPIRATION

NORMAL LARYNX: PHONATION

FIG. 16. Examination of the larynx. Copyright *Clinical Symposia* by Frank H. Netter, M.D., published by CIBA Pharmaceutical Company.

reflex can be examined directly under general anesthesia; most infants must be examined this way. A laryngoscope is used for this examination. A laryngoscope is a hollow metal tube with a distal light source illuminating the area beyond the end of the tube; different sizes and shapes are available to accommodate the size of the orifice (29, p. 142).

The patient lies on the examining table with his head beyond the end of the table; an assistant supports the head, moving it for examination procedures while another assistant handles suction apparatus (29, p. 142). DeWeese and Saunders (29, pp. 145–146) described the procedure as follows: "To do a direct examination of the larynx, the endoscopist stands above the head of the supine patient. A laryngoscope is introduced into the patient's mouth over the tongue . . . the patient's neck is slowly extended, and the laryngoscope is passed carefully over the posterior face of the epiglottis . . . to expose the vocal cords."

Radiological Examinations

Children with velopharyngeal insufficiency usually require some type of x-ray examination to determine the extent of the defect. Lateral head plates may be taken with the palate at rest and while the child sustains various sounds such as /ɑ/, /i/, and /s/. Cinefluorography, x-ray motion pictures at 24 frames per sec, may be used for a more detailed analysis of velopharyngeal function. Measurements are made of the distance between the soft palate and posterior pharyngeal wall. Generally an opening under 2 mm, measured in a lateral view, has no adverse effect on articulation or resonance. However, larger openings are acceptable for vowels preceding and following nasal sounds. Some speakers with velopharyngeal insufficiency with openings larger than 2 mm have acceptable speech and resonance. The reverse may also be true, some speakers with openings under 2 mm may have noticeable articulation or hypernasality problems. Thus when receiving reports of measurements of lateral x-ray films the speech clinician should recognize the limitations of this type of measurement.

Further guidelines for interpreting lateral x-ray reports may be helpful. Buck (21), studying a group of normal subjects, measured lateral head plates to determine the smallest velopharyngeal opening during phonation. The results were /æ/ 0.36 mm, /i/ 0.26 mm, /ɑ/ 0.15 mm, /u/ 0.12 mm. Moll (63) studied 10 adults with normal speech by cinefluorography. Measurements of velum-pharynx distance on vowels were usually zero except for vowels preceding and following /n/. The mean velum-pharynx distance on vowels preceding /n/ averaged 4.45 mm while the distance following /n/ averaged 2.15 mm.

Hagerty and Hoffmeister (40) measured velopharyngeal closure of cleft palate patients using lateral x-ray head plates. Three views were taken, the palate at rest and during the production of /ɑ/ and /s/. The measurements were related to degree of articulation problem.

Articulation Problem	Palate at Rest	/ɑ/ Sound	/s/ Sound
None	7.6 mm	2.0 mm	0.25 mm
Minor	8.6 mm	3.3 mm	2.25 mm
Moderate	9.9 mm	4.8 mm	3.50 mm
Severe	12.7 mm	10.9 mm	11.40 mm

They also presented measurements on the relationship between minimal velopharyngeal distance and nasality. They stated it is possible to predict nasality from x-rays with about 75% accuracy.

Amount of Nasality	Velopharyngeal Opening
None	0–1 mm
Minor	2–3 mm
Moderate and Severe	4 mm or more

Subtelny, Koepp-Baker, and Subtelny (99) found hypernasal speech was associated with moderate velopharyngeal openings from 3.5 to 7.0 mm.

Correlating the Voice Examination with the Physical Examination

The analysis of a child's voice should be correlated with the physical examination. Positive physical findings such as vocal nodules of a specific size and location or an inactive soft palate guide the speech clinician in his choice of examinations, in determining goals of voice therapy, and in selecting therapy measures. We can hypothesize how physiological insufficiencies and pathologies can affect the voice (109, p. 366). The reverse is true, that is, it is possible to hypothesize the physiological insufficiency or pathology according to the presenting vocal symptoms.

Arnold (4) presented some guidelines used by laryngologists. (1) The voice disorder is related to the state of the vocal cord margins. He stated, "Any irregularity of the vibrating vocal cord margin causes incomplete glottal closure." This incomplete closure results in breathiness or air escape. Arnold stressed the more marked the alterations in the edges of the vocal cords the greater the voice deviation will be usually manifesting itself in a roughness of tone. (2) The site of the lesion should be considered. The anterior-posterior position of a lesion on a vocal cord generally determines the severity of the voice problem. Lesions in the anterior commissure cause the most severe voice disorders while variations in the posterior section of the cords result in less severe vocal disturbances. (3) If there is paralytic atrophy or traumatic deficiency there will be breathiness, a waste of air, a loss of vocal intensity, and shortened phonation time.

According to Moore (65, pp. 681–682) when a speech clinician listens to vocal production the physiological condition can be hypothesized as follows.

Some weighting of the cords might be suspected as with edema or growths if the pitch is regularly very low combined with a rough hoarseness. A growth on a vocal cord such as a nodule or inadequate arytenoid approximation is suggested if the voice becomes increasingly breathy at higher pitches. One might suspect edema, growths, or inflammatory conditions producing excess mucus if the voice is hoarse at low pitches and becomes clear at high pitches. A high pitch may be due to an anterior laryngeal web or failure of laryngeal development. Baynes (6) found children with a predominately harsh voice quality had a hyperkeratotic condition while those with a breathy voice quality had a well defined pathology such as vocal nodules. Hypernasality in a child may cause the clinician to suspect velopharyngeal inadequacy or anterior growths in the nose. Hypernasality also may be the result of imitation or part of the learned pattern of speaking because of the particular region where he lives. When hyponasality is present one may suspect a partial or complete obstruction in the nasopharynx or posterior nasal passages.

The laryngologist's report must be available as the speech clinician prepares and conducts the voice examination. Special attention should be given to all physical deviations noted by the laryngologist and they should be correlated with the results of the voice examination.

The Case History

It is necessary to obtain a special case history of the child's voice and voice problem from infancy to the present. The physician and speech clinician cooperate in obtaining this information. The voice case history is designed to explore the etiology of the voice disorder as well as the factors contributing to the problem. This is in addition to a general case history which includes the general background of the child's growth and development including speech and language. Outlines for a general case history can be found in standard texts (49; 102). The suggested outline for a history of the voice problem follows.

Voice Case History Interview

Nature of Disorder. What is the parent's or patient's description of the voice disorder? How much of a problem is the disorder? Under what circumstances is it most troublesome?

Causes and Onset. What does the parent or patient regard as the cause? When was the disorder first noticed? By whom? Under what circumstances? Was its appearance sudden or gradual? Did it follow an illness?

Severity. Does the severity of the disorder vary? Describe the changes. Has it been better or worse recently? Does it vary according to the season? time of day? geographic location? weather? fatigue? mood (e.g., happiness, discouragement)?

Family History. Does any other family member have a voice, speech, or hearing problem? Does the child sound like any other family member when he talks? Does he sound like a friend or his teacher? Is his voice ever confused with anyone else on the phone? Has the child ever lived in any other part of the country? Have his parents lived elsewhere?

Voice Use. When the child was an infant did he cry and scream more than other babies? Did he have any abnormality in respiration such as noisy breathing? Has he been a noisy or talkative child? Does he yell, shout, or scream excessively when he plays? How much talking does he do when riding in a car at high speeds? How much singing does he do? Does he sing solos or in a chorus or choir? Does he participate in dramatics or cheer-leading? Does he spend much time talking in noisy places?

Medical. When was his last medical examination? What was the physician's name? What were the findings? What medications does he take regularly? List all operations and give the hospital and date for each. Has he had any serious illnesses? At what ages? Has he been in any accidents? Does he have allergies? hay fever? asthma? Does he have many colds? Has he ever had any eye trouble? Has he ever had any general breathing problems?

Has he ever had a metabolism test? If so what were the results? Was he given medication? What is his usual body temperature? Are his skin and hair dry? Does he perspire more or less than others? Do you know what his pulse rate is? Is he often fatigued without apparent cause? Has he ever been anemic? Do you know what his blood count is?

Ears. Has he been examined by an otologist? Who? Where? When? What were the findings? Has he ever had ear trouble? Injury to the ears? Operation on the ears? Has he had medical treatment for an otological problem? What are the results of any hearing tests?

Nose and Nasopharynx. Has there been injury to the nose? Has he had sinus infections? Has he ever had a deviated septum? A broken nose? Has he ever had trouble breathing through his nose, one side or both? Is he a mouth breather? Has he had difficulty with the sense of smell? Are /m/, /n/, and /ŋ/ adequately nasalized? Do they have a muffled sound? Has he ever had an adenoidectomy? Removal of nasal polyp?

Oral Cavity. Has there been injury to the mouth? Has he ever had a tonsillectomy? Has his voice been different since then? If he has had an operation on the palate why was it performed? Describe the surgery. Did it change his voice? Does he have difficulty producing speech sounds requiring oral breath pressure? Are some speech sounds emitted through the nose? What are they? Is there audible nasal emission of air as he talks? Has he ever had difficulty with the sense of taste? When he talks does he have facial grimaces or pinching of the nostrils? Has he ever had difficulty swallowing? Choking? Have liquids or food ever gone into his nose when swallowing? Can he blow up a balloon? Can he whistle? Can he drink from a fountain? With a straw?

Larynx and Hypopharynx. Has he ever been examined by a laryngologist? Who? When? Where? What were the findings? Has there been any injury to the neck? Has he ever had laryngitis? Lost his voice? Does he cough a great deal? Clear his throat often? Has there been any medical treatment for a laryngeal problem? Has there been an operation on the laryngeal area? Why was it performed? Describe the operation. Has his voice been any different since the operation? Has he ever had pain or a sense of pressure around the larynx? Is swallowing ever difficult? Does food ever lodge in the throat causing coughing?

History of Adolescence. Has the child gone through voice change? Describe the voice during this period. Describe any pitch breaks. If a girl, has she started menstruating? At what age did she begin? What is the length of the cycle? Is periodic hoarseness related to the menstrual cycle? Has the child ever worked? Was it in a noisy place? A dusty place? Does he smoke? How much? When did he start smoking?

Voice Therapy History. Has he had a previous voice or speech examination? Where? When? By whom? What were the findings? Has he had any remedial voice or speech work? What kind? Where? When? By whom? How long was it continued? Describe the results. Why was it terminated?

Examination Procedures by the Speech Clinician

The speech clinician is responsible for conducting detailed examinations of voice problems. Pitch and loudness are studied. Voice quality is defined and described as accurately as possible. Vocal abuse must be detected and evaluated. Undue muscular tensions are noted. Breathing habits are checked. Posture is noted, especially in relation to the position of the head and neck. The speech clinician may use special speech tests and oral breath pressure measures to evaluate velopharyngeal competence. The voice examination includes a brief concentrated therapy session to determine the child's ability to produce a better voice.

The assessment of vocal function is coordinated with the general physical examination, head and neck examination, psychological assessments, hearing evaluations, and other indicated examinations and tests. From the results of the examinations a plan is formulated for the voice therapy program and a prognosis of recovery potential is made.

Group Play Observation

It is necessary to obtain voice samples under various speaking conditions. Samples of voice should be obtained under two conditions, when the person knows he is being tested and when he is unaware of being tested (62, p. 301). Observations in small informal gatherings, a regular school class, and in large groups reveal use of voice (47, pp. 85–86). Many aspects of vocal behavior may not appear in a one-to-one relationship of an adult with the child. Observation of children in informal but carefully planned play situations gives excellent samples of voice use when they are unaware and when they are aware of being tested. We call this type of evaluation *group play observation*. Many times group play observation can be done by people other than the speech clinician. In a college or university it may be a student clinician, in a hospital or community clinic it may be a volunteer worker, or in the schools it may be a teacher or a teacher aide. If observers other than qualified speech clinicians are used it is necessary to instruct these assistants on observation techniques. It is not essential for the observer to be a participant in the group play situation; however, it is advisable for him to participate as much as possible to allow him to direct the activities and encourage children to talk so he can observe the various parameters of voice usage. In the Jacksonville, Florida, Child Guidance and Speech Correction Clinic on diagnostic days we used group play observation with much success to evaluate children's voices as well as other aspects of their behavior.

Group play observation can be easily set up in schools and clinics. A 45-min group play period can be scheduled. Children are grouped according to age so activities appropriate to the children's ages can be conducted. These may range from group games for nursery age children to baseball for teenagers. Children are encouraged to engage in all types of play ranging from quiet to very loud noisy activities. A relatively small room can be used for groups of three to six children. If the groups are large or if much activity is desired large rooms, gym areas, and outdoor playgrounds may be used.

Group Play Observation Form. The form to use for group play observation is shown in Figure 17. The form is based on one developed at the clinic in Jacksonville, Florida. With younger children we like to get a description of the child's behavior and attitude as he is being separated from his parents or taken from the classroom and invited to go to a playroom, a gym, or a playground. Item 1 is a description of the child's preliminary behavior and attitude. The more secure and cooperative child will easily separate from the parent or teacher. An insecure child who is reluctant to leave the parent or classroom may later present a problem in establishing rapport during voice therapy. Item 2 is a description of the child's various activities during the period, his appropriate use of toys and equipment, his need for help, his destructiveness, and his coordination. The third item deals with the child's relationship to adults and to other children. Item 4, the level of the child's operation, may reveal information about his learning ability. The observer may note under Item 5 the child's

Name_____ Birth Date_____ Age_____

Place of observation: Playroom, gym, playground, other_____

Observer_____ Date_____ Length of Observation_____

1. Describe preliminary behavior and attitude.

2. Describe activities in which the child engaged, appropriate use of toys, equipment, need for help, destructiveness, coordination.

3. Relationships to adults and other children.

4. Learning ability: Level of operation observed.

5. Hearing: Response to noise and speech.

6. Speech: Amount, intelligibility, rhythm, use of gestures to communicate, estimate of language ability.

7. Voice: Pitch, loudness, quality; do these aspects vary under different conditions? Voice breaks, monotone.

8. Vocal abuse: Shouting, screaming, cheering, strained vocalizations, excessive talking, reverse phonation, explosive release of vocalizations, abrupt glottal attack, throat clearing, coughing.

9. Overall impression of the child, including speech and voice.

10. Recommendations:

FIG. 17. Group play observation.

responses to noise and speech which reveal information about his listening abilities.

Items 6 and 7 are concerned specifically with a child's speech and voice. Careful observations should be made of the amount of talking, intelligibility of speech, rhythm of speech, use of gestures to communicate, and general language ability. The observer should listen very carefully to the child's voice. The pitch of his voice should be noted. Is it appropriate to his age and sex? What happens to it when the voice increases in loudness? Does the pitch rise appropriately as loudness increases? What is the general level of loudness? How much loud talking does he do? Is the quality of his voice hypernasal, hyponasal, breathy, harsh, or hoarse? If any differences in pitch, loudness, or quality have been noted the observer should listen carefully to see if these deviations vary under different conditions. For example, what happens to a hoarse voice with an increase in loudness? Does the quality get worse or does it seem to clear up? Any voice breaks and monotonous use of voice in the group play situation should be noted.

Item 8, vocal abuse, is a particularly important item in group play observation. Various types of vocal abuse to be noted include shouting, screaming, cheering, excessive talking, strained vocalization, reverse phonation, explosive release of vocalizations, abrupt glottal attack, throat clearing, and coughing. Definitions of these were given in Chapter 2. The observation form also includes the observer's overall impression of the child and recommendations for special testing based on the observation.

Voice Rating Scales

The speech clinician uses rating scales to evaluate voice in its various parameters. Each child is rated to establish baselines of vocal behavior.

Establishing Baselines

Baselines are descriptions of behavior a person exhibits. Rating scales can be used to describe such behavior. A child's use of voice is rated before any treatment is started to enable the clinician to know the level of vocal behavior and the aspects which should be improved.

Behavior must be correctly identified and reliably measured (20). Therefore, the speech clinician in measuring any type of vocal behavior or speech behavior for establishing baselines must be sure the measurements are consistently and reliably made. Our examination and evaluative procedures include establishment of baselines for deviant voice behavior through the use of rating scales such as the rating of vocal abuse practices. Brookshire (20) emphasized the necessity for establishing baselines in varying situations. For example, some children may shout only to a moderate degree in one situation, while in another situation shouting may be extremely loud, and in still other situations he may not shout at all.

Brookshire (20) pointed out the establishment of specific baselines and their exact identification and measurement "...forces the clinician to define specific observable behaviors of concern prior to initiation of therapy." These baselines then become the foundation from which improvement can be measured as therapy progresses with final ratings made at the conclusion of therapy. These final ratings are compared with ratings made when children are seen for follow-up evaluations to check effectiveness of carryover.

Rating Scales

The equal-appearing intervals rating scale is the most frequently used scale in speech pathology. Sherman and Moodie (93) compared four different methods of scaling articulation defectiveness of children's speech and found the method of equal-appearing intervals to be most satisfactory. We recommend the use of this type of scale for voice evaluations. This scale usually includes three to seven points. A disadvantage of the equal-appearing intervals scale is called the "end effect" (26), that is a judge's tendency to refrain from using the extreme ends of a scale. The speech clinician should keep this tendency in mind and use the end ratings whenever indicated.

To be a reliable and valid rater a judge has to be trained specifically for that task. Having experience in speech and voice therapy is not sufficient background for precise judging of voice. Villarreal (105) found a low percentage of agreement among judges in rating voice quality. Bradford, Brooks, and Shelton (13) also found unreliable ratings were made by both inexperienced and experienced speech clinicians who were not comprehensively trained specifically for the task of rating hypernasality. Thus speech clinicians should prove their competency in judging various aspects of voice. This can be done through judging types and severity of voice deviations and correlating the ratings with those of other clinicians. Reliability or consistency in rating can be determined by comparing the results of periodic ratings of the same samples.

The number of intervals used on a scale is determined by the characteristics and complexities of the item to be rated. For example, three points can be used for some scales while more points are desirable for others. Three points can be used in describing the amount of certain vocal characteristics such as shouting, with *1* meaning little shouting, *2* frequent shouting, and *3* excessive shouting. Three points are also satisfactory for rating the degree of vocal effort. For example, rating throat clearing can be done with *1* indicating a mild degree of effort or force, *2* a moderate degree, or *3* a severe degree, that is very hard, forceful, and loud throat clearing. In rating other vocal attributes, hoarseness for example, it is desirable to use a seven point scale with *1* indicating a slight deviation and *7* a severe deviation

General Voice Profile

A general voice profile is used in rating a voice problem and as a guideline for voice therapy (Fig. 18). Special rating scales for specific voice problems are also used and will be presented later. The scales of the general voice profile contain seven equal-appearing intervals with *1* meaning a slight deviation and *7* a severe deviation. This profile consists of ten major aspects: pitch, vocal inflections, laryngeal tone, laryngeal tension, vocal abuse, resonance, nasal emission, loudness, rate, and overall voice efficiency. The speech clinician circles the appropriate descriptive term listed under each item. For example, pitch may be rated as normal, high, or low. If pitch is rated normal it requires no further rating. If it is rated either high or low the clinician must circle one of the numbers on the deviation scale for that item. He should not place checks between the numbers. The same procedure is used for all ten items.

Name_____ Birth Date_____ Age_____ Sex_____

Rater_____ Date_____ Time of Day_____ Place_____

1. PITCH
Normal
High   1   2   3   4   5   6   7
Low

2. VOCAL INFLECTIONS
Normal
Monotone   1   2   3   4   5   6   7
Excessive

3. LARYNGEAL TONE
Normal
Breathy
Harsh   1   2   3   4   5   6   7
Hoarse

4. LARYNGEAL TENSION
Normal
Hypertense   1   2   3   4   5   6   7
Hypotense

5. VOCAL ABUSE
No
Yes   1   2   3   4   5   6   7

6. RESONANCE
Normal
Hypernasal   1   2   3   4   5   6   7
Hyponasal

7. NASAL EMISSION
No
Yes   1   2   3   4   5   6   7

8. LOUDNESS
Normal
Too Loud   1   2   3   4   5   6   7
Too Soft

9. RATE
Normal
Fast   1   2   3   4   5   6   7
Slow

10. OVERALL VOICE EFFICIENCY
Adequate   1   2   3   4   5   6   7
Inadequate

COMMENTS:

INSTRUCTIONS:
   A. Circle the appropriate descriptive term under *each* item.
   B. For each item *not* normal or adequate, circle a number on the scale for that item.
      Do *not* mark between numbers.
     Key: 1 = slight deviation   7 = severe deviation

Fig. 18. General voice profile.

Types of Voice Samples

In studying the various aspects of voice the speech clinician should obtain several types of speech samples. These samples should include connected speech, oral reading, isolated speech sounds, and counting. All samples of voice or speech should be tape recorded for further use and study.

Connected Speech. A sample of connected speech can usually be obtained by asking the child to tell a story about a picture. Action pictures of various types can be used to obtain such samples. Wilson (115) found the picture from the Myklebust Picture Story Language Test (73) useful for this purpose. Another way to get samples of connected speech is to ask questions about a specific topic such as a trip with the family.

Oral Reading. If the child is old enough to read, it is desirable to get an oral reading sample. For children of approximately third grade reading level and above we use a passage which we devised several years ago titled "The Trip to the Zoo." The same passage should be used for all children old enough to read so when listening judgments are made the speech clinician is not distracted by an unfamiliar passage but can concentrate on evaluating the voice and its attributes. For this reason this same passage should be used when checking progress in voice therapy. If the child's reading level is below third grade his own reading book should be used to get as smooth a sample of reading as possible.

The Trip to the Zoo

Last Sunday Bob went to the zoo with his mother and father. His sister Mary and his brother George went along too. Mother packed a big basket full of good things to eat. Father took the car to the service station to get gas and to have the oil checked. The family left the house at 11 o'clock and got to the zoo at 12 o'clock. You can see that they didn't have far to go.

At the zoo they saw monkeys, tigers, lions, bears, elephants, and lots of beautiful birds. The monkeys put on a special show in their cage. They jumped from one swing to another and pulled each other around in little red wagons. The elephants put on a show too. They stood up on their hind legs and danced with each other.

After the shows the family found a nice cool place under a tree. Mother put a table cloth on the grass and unpacked the lunch. The family ate the lunch and talked about the good time they had seeing all the animals at the zoo.

Isolated Speech Sounds. A sample of isolated vowel production should be obtained. All of the long vowels (/e/, /i/, /aɪ/, /o/, /u/) and short vowels (/æ/, /ɛ/, /ɪ/, /ɑ/, /ʌ/) should be used paying particular attention to long vowels which are more easily sustained. Selected voiced continuant consonants, for example /m/, /n/, /r/, /l/, should also be recorded. Each sound should be rated on a three point scale, with *1* a mild deviation, *2* moderate, and *3* severe. Except for short vowels each sound should be sustained for at least 5 sec for careful study.

We usually find some sounds have little or no voice deviation while others have much deviation. Van Riper (102, p. 470) stated, "All vowels are seldom equally bad, and usually only a few need remedial work." Voice training can begin by comparing sounds which are relatively clear and free of the undesirable voice quality with those sounds that have a significant amount of vocal deviation.

It is profitable to compare a child's voice quality on sustained isolated vowels with the results of certain research studies. Although these studies were done on adults we are applying them to children. Research results do not always coincide or agree exactly but the findings indicate a tendency for some vowels to be more harsh or hoarse than others. For example, Sherman and Linke (92) found that a passage containing mainly the high vowels /i/, /u/, /ɪ/, /ʊ/ was perceived by the judges as *less harsh* than a passage with low vowels /æ/, /ɔ/, and /ɑ/. The passage with lax vowels /ɪ/, /ʊ/, /ɛ/, /æ/, /ɑ/ was perceived as *less harsh* than the one containing tense vowels, /i/, /u/, /e/, /o/, and /ɔ/.

Rees (83) analyzed hoarseness on vowels. Her results indicated the following order from least harsh to most harsh /i/, /u/, /ɪ/, /ʊ/, /ʌ/, /ɛ/, /æ/, /ɑ/, and /ɔ/. This corresponds closely to Sherman and Linke's comparison of high and low vowels. Yanagihara (118) in a sound spectrographic study of hoarseness found noise elements more evident in the vowels /ɑ/, /ɛ/, and /i/ than in the vowels /u/ and /ɔ/.

We use a practical test based upon Yanagihara's (118) findings. We follow his instructions by asking the child first to glide from /u/ to /i/ and then sustain each of the five vowels used in his study for at least 5 sec. The speech clinician listens carefully to any additional noise components heard as the child performs. Noise components may be heard as breathiness, harshness, or hoarseness present during voiced sound production. Some vowels will have additional noise components; others may be quite free of the noise components. These are rated on the scale from one to three. Rating laryngeal tone according to amount of noise components heard is a useful test once the speech clinician becomes experienced with this type of rating. The child's performance on vowels furnishes material for discrimination training.

Counting. It is desirable to record a child counting from 1 to 10. Have him count twice, first slowly and carefully and then again as rapidly as possible but still saying each number carefully. This should be done under three levels of loudness: soft, average, and loud. The contrast between the countings may exaggerate or even reveal pitch and loudness misuse, vocal abuse, defective laryngeal tone, or resonance problems.

Effect of Stimulation

Another important step in the analysis of quality disorders is to determine the effect of specific stimulation on voice quality. Van Riper (102, pp. 470–471) listed several types of stimulation as follows. Use two or three of the most deviant sounds and vary the position of the tongue and lips to see if this results in improved quality. These same deviant sounds can be used to investigate the effect of different pitch levels on the quality of the voice. This can be tried with continuous speech as well as isolated vowels. The same sort of trial can be made by varying the loudness of the voice to determine whether a louder voice or a softer voice reveals better quality. Sometimes when a child imitates someone with a good voice he will sound a little better. Van Riper and Irwin (104, p. 282) suggested noting differences in voice quality when a child sings and hums. Thus, through these types of stimulation we find those sounds and situations in which the voice quality is at its worst and those in which it is at its best.

Analysis of Pitch and Loudness

Many times it is necessary to teach children to use pitch levels which are adequate and nontraumatizing; therefore, it is necessary to make a careful analysis of the child's use of pitch and loudness before planning voice therapy. This includes determining habitual pitch and comparing it to standards for his age and sex.

When examining a child's use of pitch he should be observed under various voice intensity conditions. We know pitch becomes higher with an increase in the intensity of a person's voice from normal to loud; likewise, a lowering of pitch occurs when a person goes from normal to soft speech. A study of a child's pitch when talking at loud levels may reveal information on the misuse of the vocal mechanism.

The study of a child's pitch should be made with knowledge of the results of his laryngeal examination. The pitch level used by children with certain pathologies such as vocal nodules may be quite crucial. If the habitual pitch is too high it should lowered because such pitch misuse is sometimes a contributing factor in the formation of vocal nodules. A detailed pitch analysis may not be necessary if pitch usage seems appropriate and there are no laryngeal pathologies thought to be connected with pitch use. There is no need to be unnecessarily preoccupied with pitch manipulation (17).

Pitch Analysis

Pitch analysis can be made using a musical instrument, pitch pipe, or pitch meter. A piano, guitar, or other musical instrument can be used. However, many times a musical instrument is not available and a pitch pipe may not have enough notes to give variety and range to the study of a child's use of pitch. Instruments for pitch analysis in the clinical situation are available.* With this type of instrument the speech clinician does not have to be familiar with the musical scale to determine the child's habitual pitch. The child's use of pitch inflections can be studied using a pitch meter. Direct readings in Hertz can be obtained from the VU meter on the front of the instrument. Some instruments are designed to use lights to indicate correct and incorrect use of pitch.†

The habitual pitch level can be determined with a pitch meter following Fairbanks' technique (31, p. 126). Give the child a reading selection of about 180 words. Place vertical lines after about the first 60 words and the second set of 60 words. Have the child read the first third of the passage with normal inflections. When he reaches the first pair of vertical lines have him begin to compress his range gradually until he is chanting in a monotone at his habitual pitch level by the time he reaches the second pair of vertical lines. Let him finish the third section of the passage on this pitch gradually changing to humming or singing the note equal to his pitch level. For younger children who cannot read fluently have them repeat a familiar nursery rhyme or poem several times. Hand gestures can be used to signal for compression of pitch. During this process the clinician watches the pitch meter readings carefully, finally ending up with a definite reading during the third section of the reading passage. As the child compresses his pitch the needle on the pitch meter will barely fluctuate. The average of the observable fluctuations will be the habitual pitch level. The whole procedure should be repeated several times to determine accuracy of measurements. The same method can be used with a piano or musical instrument. Next compare the pitch meter readings or the musical note for his habitual pitch with the acceptable limits for his age (Tables 2 and 3).

Basic Pitch Abilities. If we decide to change the child's habitual pitch level, Van Riper (102, pp. 467–468) recommended determining a child's basic pitch abilities as follows. (1) Assess the child's ability to discriminate pitch. The speech clinician hums, whistles, or sings pairs of notes one tone apart to see if the child can determine if the first note is higher or lower. (2) Check the child's ability to imitate a given pitch. The speech clinician hums at various pitches (low, middle, and high) and asks the child to match the tones. (3) See if the child can carry a simple tune either in unison or alone. (4) Test the child's ability to follow upward and downward inflections. If the child performs poorly on these tasks he will need a concentrated program in pitch discrimination.

---

* PAD pitch meter, Datac, Inc., Cleveland, Ohio, 44118. Fundamental Frequency Indicator, Special Instrument, Stockholm, Sweden. United States Distributor: 410 Overland Drive, Chapel Hill, North Carolina 27514.

† Florida I, Saber, Inc., Cocoa Beach, Florida 32931 (controls both pitch and loudness levels).

TABLE 2

Composite Pitch Chart—Boys

Age	Fundamental Frequency	Acceptable Limits of Fundamental Frequency	Nearest Musical Note to Fundamental Frequency	Acceptable Limits of Fundamental Frequency in Musical Notes
	Hz	*Hz*		
1 & 2	*445*	*370–525*	A_4	$F\#_4–C_5$
3	400	340–460	G_4	$F_4–A\#_4$
4	375	320–425	$F\#_4$	$D\#_4–G\#_4$
5	350	300–390	F_4	$D_4–G_4$
6	325	280–365	E_4	$C\#_4–F\#_4$
7	*295*	*260–330*	D_4	$C_4–E_4$
8	*295*	*260–330*	D_4	$C_4–E_4$
9	260	220–300	C_4	$A_3–D_4$
10	*235*	*195–275*	$A\#_3$	$G_3–C\#_4$
11	225	185–260	A_3	$F\#_3–C_4$
12	210	170–245	$G\#_3$	$F_3–B_3$
13	195	155–230	G_3	$D\#_3–A\#_3$
14	*190*	*155–220*	$F\#_3$	$D\#_3–A_3$
15	165	130–195	E_3	$C_3–G_3$
16	150	120–180	D_3	$A\#_2–F\#_3$
17	135	110–170	$C\#_3$	$A_2–F_3$
18	*125*	*100–155*	B_2	$G_2–D\#_3$

The pitch charts (Tables 2 and 3), including all ages, are presented to give the speech clinician standards to use in checking the appropriateness of a child's habitual pitch. The pitch charts are based upon the research studies given in Table 4. The *italicized figures* in the pitch charts are from the research studies. The fundamental frequency is either that in the one study in Table 4 for that age or an average of the fundamental frequencies in all the studies for that age. The figures in regular type present values hypothesized by drawing curves of best fit according to inspection. The pitch charts were devised for use with either a pitch meter or musical instrument. Column 1 lists the ages; Column 2, the fundamental frequency in Hertz; Column 3, the acceptable limits of the fundamental frequency in Hertz; Column 4, the nearest musical note to the fundamental frequency; and Column 5, the acceptable limits of the fundamental frequency in musical notes. Fundamental frequencies and acceptable limits in Hertz were rounded to the nearest 5 Hz for convenience in using a pitch meter. The Westphal Chart (110) was used in establishing relationships between musical notes and Hertz values.

Mutation. When examining an adolescent the speech clinician should note mutational changes in the voice. A boy's voice may lower as much as an octave during the period of mutation and a girl's voice may lower 2 or 3 semitones. During mutational changes huskiness or excessive voice

TABLE 3

Composite Pitch Chart—Girls

Age	Fundamental Frequency	Acceptable Limits of Fundamental Frequency	Nearest Musical Note to Fundamental Frequency	Acceptable Limits of Fundamental Frequency in Musical Notes
	Hz	*Hz*		
1 & 2	*445*	*370–525*	A_4	$F\#_4$–C_5
3	380	335–475	$F\#_4$	E_4–$A\#_4$
4	355	310–450	F_4	$D\#_4$–A_4
5	335	290–425	E_4	D_4–$G\#_4$
6	315	270–395	$D\#_4$	$C\#_4$–G_4
7	*280*	*245–310*	$C\#_4$	B_3–$D\#_4$ $(F_4)^a$
8	*290*	*245–350*	D_4	B_3–F_4
9	275	235–335	$C\#_4$	$A\#_3$–E_4
10	265	225–320	C_4	A_3–$D\#_4$
11	*265*	*220–310*	C_4	A_3–$D\#_4$
12	260	220–310	C_4	$G\#_3$–D_4
13I[b]	*260*	*235–295*	C_4	$A\#_3$–D_4
13II[b]	*245*	*210–295*	B_3	$G\#_3$–D_4
14	235	195–270	$A\#_3$	G_3–$C\#_4$
15	*220*	*185–260*	A_3	$F\#_3$–C_4
16	*215*	*185–260*	A_3	$F\#_3$–C_4
17	*210*	*175–245*	$G\#_3$	F_3–B_3
18	205	175–245	$G\#_3$	F_3–B_3

[a] Preferred upper limit.
[b] 13I = premenarche; 13II = postmenarche.

breaks may be noted. However, voice breaks may appear in both girls and boys as young as 7 or 8 years of age (32; 33).

A practical test to use on male adolescents with delayed or incomplete mutation is Gutzmann's (39) pressure test as described by Brodnitz (15). This test is especially useful in psychogenic mutational voice problems. Ordinarily, pressure on the thyroid cartilage during phonation produces an initial lowering of pitch in the normal voice. Brodnitz, however, found in psychogenic falsetto voices, pressure on the thyroid cartilage produced an initial pitch rise instead of the usual lowering. With training such cases usually begin to show the ordinary response of a lowering of the pitch of the voice with pressure on the thyroid cartilage.

Loudness Analysis

How loud should a child talk? He should talk loud enough to be heard according to the situation and the background noise but not so loud as to be unpleasant to listeners. Rubin (85) indicated the use of excessive volume over a prolonged period of time has a detrimental effect even when the voice is used efficiently. When loudness control is a problem the results of the hearing evaluation should be reviewed.

TABLE 4

Pitch Table: Results of Research

Age	Fundamental Frequency[a] Hz	Standard Deviation in Tones	Number of Subjects	Reference
		Males		
1 & 2	443.3	1.70	6	59
7	294	1.1	15	33
8	297	1.0	15	33
10	263.5	1.19	6	27
	210.2	1.90	6	43
	235.4	1.48	6	45
	226.4	1.82	6	44
14	232.7	1.70	6	27
	158.2	1.20	6	43
	185.8	1.66	6	45
	184	1.32	6	44
18	133.1	1.79	6	27
	121.9	1.42	6	43
	115.9	2.21	6	45
		Females		
1 & 2	443.3	1.70	6	59
7	281	1.0	15	32
8	288	1.4	15	32
11	266	1.34	6	30
13I	260	1.22	6	30
13II	245	1.72	6	30
15	237	1.33	6	30
	215.7	1.53	89	61; 46
16	213.9	1.48	185	61; 46
17	211.5	1.67	193	61; 46

[a] Note: All fundamental frequencies are means. Means for References 27 and 43 were obtained from Reference 45. Data from Reference 59 included both males and females. In Reference 30, 13I indicates premenarche and 13II postmenarche.

The following studies were done with adults, but until there is more information on the loudness ranges and levels of children's voices we will make inferences from these studies. The measurement values vary according to the distance of the speaker from the sound level meter. Fletcher (34, pp. 76–77) stated the range of face-to-face speech at a distance of 40 inches is 46 to 86 dB. Black (10) defined the range from soft to loud speech as spanning about 30 dB, that is, about 70 dB for soft speech to 100 dB for loud speech at a distance of 18 inches from a sound level meter. Yanagihara, Koike, and von Leden (120) measured vocal intensity of adults when the microphone was approximately 8 inches from the outlet of a ρneumotach tube attached to a facial mask. The average vocal intensity of the male subjects was 67 dB and for females 64 dB.

Subjective estimates of the loudness of a child's voice can be made as he engages in various activities ranging from relatively inactive play to very active play. Van Riper and Irwin (104, p. 282) suggested the clinician note the loudness level in the expression of emotion and during various kinds of physical activities. If a sound level meter is available objective measurements of the loudness of a child's voice can be made. However, most loudness evaluations are made subjectively and rated on the voice profile. Attention to the loudness level should be incorporated into the voice therapy program if parents, teachers, and the speech clinician agree a child has an excessively loud or soft manner of talking.

Measurement of Phonation Time

A child should have an adequate supply of air and be able to maintain steady phonation sufficient for effective speech communication. The measurement of maximum phonation time is an index of this ability. Research has been conducted on maximum phonation time of adults and children. Ptacek and Sander (81) using 40 men and 40 women, found the maximum phonation time for men averaged about 25 sec and for women about 17 sec. Yanagihara et al. (120) and Yanagihara and Koike (119) measured maximum phonation time in normal adults. Phonation time was reported at three different vocal pitches, low, medium, and high. Phonation time was reduced at high pitch levels for both men and women. The figures for men were 28.4 sec for low pitch, 30.2 sec for medium pitch, and 23.7 sec for high pitch. The figures for women were 21.7 sec for low pitch, 22.5 sec for medium pitch, and 16.7 sec for high pitch. Launer (52) measured maximum phonation time for /ɑ/, /i/, and /u/ on 179 children (95 females and 84 males) aged 9 through 17 years. There were no statistically significant differences between the three vowels. Phonation time increased with age increase and boys had longer sustained phonation time than girls. Averaged phonation times, averaged standard deviations for the three vowels, and the number of children in each age group are shown in Table 5.

A significant reduction below normal levels can be related to inadequate voice production. Sawashima et al. (89) cited Sawashima's (88) study published in the *Japanese Journal of Lcgcpedics and Phoniatrics* showing that phonation lengths below 15 sec in adult males and below 10 sec in adult females should be regarded as pathological.

To measure maximum phonation time have the child practice sustaining the vowels /ɑ/, /i/, or /u/ at constant pitch and loudness levels. Be sure he takes a deep breath before sustaining a vowel. Then use a stop watch to time him during three sustained phonations of the vowel. Timing begins

TABLE 5

Averaged Maximum Phonation Time in Sec for /ɑ/, /i/, and /u/

Adapted from Launer, P. G. Unpublished master's thesis, State University of New York at Buffalo, 1971.

Age	Females			Males		
	Time	S.D.	N	Time	S.D.	N
	sec			sec		
9	8.8	3.6	8	11.4	5.9	5
10	9.4	2.8	7	10.4	4.2	7
11	11.5	2.7	8	12.8	7.2	8
12	12.2	3.7	9	12.2	5.3	13
13	11.0	3.5	11	12.3	4.4	15
14	13.3	6.2	12	17.6	7.2	11
15	12.4	5.2	20	18.9	6.0	10
16	12.9	2.9	10	17.8	4.5	6
17	13.5	2.9	10	16.9	8.0	9

with the initiation of phonation and ends when his voice drops to a whisper. Following is an example of a child with inadequate respiratory function.

An 8-year-old girl suffered brain damage as a result of an automobile accident. Her respiratory function was reduced so she had insufficient air flow for phonation. The first task of the speech clinician was to develop sustained phonation ability. Initially, even after many attempts, she was able to sustain phonation for only 2 or 3 sec. After 3 weeks of voice therapy with a coordinated program in physical therapy her maximum phonation time had increased to approximately 10 sec. Breathing exercises and a modified version of Froeschels' pushing technique (see Chapter 5) were used to increase phonation time and improve the quality of phonation.

Analysis of Breathing Habits

In most instances it is not necessary to evaluate breathing habits of children with voice disorders. No two persons breathe exactly alike and we should not attempt to force a universal pattern of breathing on everyone (18, p. 97). A brief analysis of breathing to make sure proper breathing is being used during speaking is usually all that is necessary. In most cases if a person can breathe adequately for physiological purposes breathing during phonation is normal. We do not need a large supply of air or high subglottic air pressure to initiate and maintain adequate vocalization (28, p. 196). However, it is necessary to analyze breathing habits for special types of voice problems such as a child with cerebral palsy (71, p. 97) or cases of extremely inefficient respiratory habits. Attention should be paid to breathing if there is something unusual about a child's physiological breathing habits, for example excessive tension of muscles or clavicular expansion (78, pp. 868–869). Abnormal breathing habits during speaking should also be noted. A child with improper breathing habits affecting his voice should be referred for medical consulation.

Examination of Resonance

Children and adolescents who have defects of resonance should be given special tests by the speech clinician before a remedial voice program is planned. Two types of problems are of interest here: hypernasality, which is most noticeable on consonants requiring high oral breath pressure and vowels, and hyponasality specifically on the /m/, /n/, and /ŋ/ sounds. Examinations for resonance problems by the speech clinician include: (1) ratings of various parameters of resonance using a resonance profile, (2) special articulation tests, and (3) oral pressure measurements.

Resonance Profile

The resonance profile (Fig. 19) is used as a supplement to the general voice profile. The directions for using this special profile are similar to the general voice profile. The speech clinician first determines whether the voice is hypernasal (Item 1) or hyponasal (Item 2) remembering, however, both characteristics can be present in one person. If so, ratings are made on both items.

On the appropriate scale the clinician then rates the defective resonance with *1* indicating a slight deviation and *7* a severe deviation. The defective sounds reflecting the resonance problem are listed. The severity of nasal emission of sounds (Item 3) is rated on the seven point scale and the sounds nasally emitted are listed. Item 4 deals with facial grimaces which usually are seen in constrictive action of the nares and occur in using words which require increased oral breath pressure (84). Facial grimaces are rated on a seven point scale and a description of the grimaces included. Item 5 is used to rate articulation defectiveness and to list defective sounds other than those listed under other items.

Articulation Tests for Hypernasality

Children with hypernasality should be given special articulation tests to determine adequacy of velopharyngeal closure (70). Shelton, Brooks, and Youngstrom (91) evaluated several methods used to measure velopharyngeal closure in children. They concluded a carefully administered articulation test is a better measure of palatopharyngeal adequacy than simple measures of nasal air escape or oral breath pressure.

The results of the articulation tests will answer Morris and Smith's (69) questions about the speech production of a person with a velopharyngeal

Name_____ Birth Date_____ Age_____ Sex_____
Rater_____ Date_____ Time of Day_____ Place_____

1. *Hypernasality*   1   2   3   4   5   6   7
   No
   Yes
   Hypernasal sounds   _____

2. *Hyponasality*   1   2   3   4   5   6   7
   No
   Yes
   Hyponasal sounds   _____

3. *Nasal Emission of Sounds*   1   2   3   4   5   6   7
   No
   Yes
   Sounds Emitted   _____

4. *Facial Grimaces* (including   1   2   3   4   5   6   7
   nares constriction)
   No
   Yes
   Describe_____

5. *Articulation Defectiveness*   1   2   3   4   5   6   7
   List defective sounds (in addition to those listed above).

Instructions:
  A. Circle the appropriate descriptive term under each item.
  B. For each item *not* normal or adequate, circle a number on the scale for that item.
     Do *not* mark between numbers.
    Key: 1 = slight deviation   7 = severe deviation
  C. List sounds where indicated.

FIG. 19. Resonance profile.

insufficiency, "Does the speaker misarticulate those consonants . . . [fricatives: /s/, /z/, /ʃ/, /f/; plosives: /k/, /g/, /t/, /d/, /p/, /b/; affricate: /dʒ/] . . . which have been demonstrated to require high intraoral breath pressure? Do the misarticulations . . . involve audible nasal emission? Are there evidences of facial contortion during the production of these consonants? Does occluding the nostrils (preventing an air leakage) result in normal production of them?"

A standard articulation test and the Iowa Pressure Articulation Test (70; 101) should both be given. The latter test consists of 43 words containing sounds which require oral pressure for correct production and discriminates between speakers who have adequate velopharyngeal closure and those who do not. The number of errors reflects the severity of the velopharyngeal incompetence. A list of the test words with the test sounds in decreasing order of their importance in discriminating between good and poor velopharyngeal closure is shown in Figure 20. The mean scores for the 43-item test are shown in Table 6. The articulation tests should include checking the child's responses to stimulation, both auditory and visual, on all sounds incorrectly produced on the tests. The amount of improvement reveals the potential for adequate velopharyngeal closure for speech (69).

The reading passage "The Picnic" using the 43 words from the Iowa Pressure Articulation Test should be recorded. In this way the production of the test words in reading can be evaluated. The test words are in *italics*.

The Picnic

Mother told the *twins*, Jimmy and Susie, to *jump* out of bed and get dressed. Mother and Susie wore pink *dresses*. Jimmy lost one *shoe* and both *socks* as he came down the *stairs*. Mother put clothes in the *washer*. The children brought *string*, *scissors*, *paper*, and *crayons*. *Two blocks* from home they saw a circus parade. A *tiger* and a *wolf* were in cages on a *wagon*. A *clown* rode in a funny *truck*. Whenever he *stopped* he ate a *cracker* and *smoke* came out of his *pocket*. A *girl* clown talks on a *telephone* and *stamps* her feet in time with a *drum*. Another clown on *skates* looks like a *snowman* wearing *glasses*. Mother gave everyone *dishes* and a *knife*, *spoon*, *fork*, *bread*, and *fish*. They sat in the *sun* and saw men *planting grass*. They saw a *cat* run after a *mouse*, and a *dog* chase a *'possum* up a *tree*.

Hypernasality on vowels should also be checked. Spriestersbach and Powers (97) had judges rate on a seven point equal-appearing intervals scale the amount of hypernasality on certain vowels in children with cleft palate speech. The vowels from *least nasal* to *most nasal* were: /ɑ/, /ʌ/, /æ/, /o/, /ɛ/, /u/, and /i/. Lintz and Sherman (55) studied nasality on vowels of adults with functional hypernasality, having judges rate the nasality in a manner similar to Spriestersbach and Powers. A somewhat different order was found from *least nasal* to *most nasal:* /u/, /ʊ/, /ʌ/, /i/, /ɛ/, /ɑ/, and /æ/. The differences in results of the two studies probably were due to different causes of the hypernasality and the different ages of the groups. Lintz and Sherman found certain consonant environments tended to influence the amount of nasality rated on vowels. From *least* influence to *most* influence were /z/, /v/, /d/, /g/, /f/, /s/, /t/, and /k/. It would seem, therefore, that nasality on vowels should be studied in these consonant environments.

Bloomer and Wolski (12) suggested obtaining samples of sounds, words, or sentences not containing /m/, /n/, or /ŋ/. For example, have the child say "Buy baby a bib," "Zippers are easy to close," "Go get a bigger egg," the numbers 2, 3, 4, 5, 6, or /i-o/ (12). Each sample should be said under

DISCRIMINATION

LEVELS	*SOUNDS*	*WORDS*
1	/s-, sk-/	*s*un, *sk*ates
2	/-k-, sm-, -sm, sn-, str-/	po*ck*et, *sm*oke, po*ss*um, *sn*owman, *str*ing
3	/ʃ-, -z-, -kɚ, st-/	*sh*oe, *s*cissors, cra*ck*er, *st*airs
4	/-s-, -ʃ-, kr-/	dre*ss*es, di*sh*es, *cr*ayons
5	/-g-, -s, sp-, tr-, gr-, -gɚ, -ɚk, -pt, kl-, gl-, -mps/	wa*g*on, mou*s*e, *sp*oon *tr*ee, *gr*ass, ti*g*er *f*or*k*, sto*pp*ed, *cl*own *gl*asses, sta*mps*
6	/k-, g-, -g, -ʃ, dʒ-, -ʃɚ, bl-, -ks/	*c*at, *g*irl, do*g*, fi*sh*, *j*ump, wa*sh*er *bl*ocks, so*cks*
7	/-k, br-, dr-, tw-/	tru*ck*, *br*ead, *dr*um, *tw*ins
8	/t-, f-, -f, -pɚ, pl-, -lf/	*t*wo, tele*ph*one, kni*f*e, pa*p*er, *pl*anting, wo*lf*

Key: Level 1 most discriminating, Level 8 least discriminating. Sounds are shown according to position in word, e.g. initial /s-/, medial/-s-/, and final /-s/.

FIG. 20. Iowa pressure articulation test sounds and words in order of decreasing discrimination levels. Discrimination levels from Morris, Spriestersbach, and Darley (70). Words from Templin and Darley (101).

TABLE 6

Mean Scores on 43-Item Iowa Pressure Articulation Test by Age for Boys and Girls

From Templin, M. C., and Darley, F. L. *The Templin-Darley Tests of Articulation —A Manual and Discussion of Articulation Testing.* Ed. 2. Iowa City: Bureau of Educational Research and Service, University of Iowa, 1969.

Age	Boys (*N* = 30)		Girls (*N* = 30)	
	Mean	S.D.	Mean	S.D.
3	26.4	12.5	23.6	11.6
3½	28.8	12.5	32.9	9.6
4	35.1	9.7	33.5	8.8
4½	34.1	9.4	35.0	8.8
5	33.8	11.2	37.5	8.6
6	35.5	10.3	39.5	6.5
7	39.6	5.7	41.6	3.0
8	42.0	3.3	41.7	2.9

two conditions, with the nares unoccluded and then occluded. Any nasal resonance present will be exaggerated on the occluded performance because of the cul-de-sac effect. With normal velopharyngeal functioning the resonance on both productions will be normal.

The speech sample should include a study of sound confusions often found in cases of velopharyngeal insufficiency. Shupe (94) used the following words in studying sound confusions in cleft palate subjects: bake/make, rib/rim, dine/nine, mad/man, wig/wing, and bag/bang. In a person with velopharyngeal insufficiency both sounds are hypernasal; for example, the bake/make pair sounds like make/make. Following is an example of submucous cleft palate.

Sharon, a 6½-year-old first grader, was brought to the speech clinic by her mother because she had a severe articulation problem and according to the mother, "Talks like she has a cleft palate." These problems had always been present but a recent head and neck examination had not been done. A tonsillectomy and adeonoidectomy were performed when she was 4½ years of age because of repeated ear infections and the operation had no adverse effect on voice resonance. The child's general health was good.

The speech examination confirmed the mother's description of speech as resembling that of a child with cleft palate. Hypernasality was present on vowels and nasal emission of air occurred on the stop sounds /p/, /b/, /t/, /d/, /k/, /g/, and on most fricative sounds including /f/, /s/, /z/, and /ʃ/. Nasality was rated *6* on a seven point scale, nasal emission *5*, and intelligibility *4*.

An examination of the oral cavity revealed a palatal condition often found in those with a submucous cleft. There was a midline notching of the uvula which looked as if it had been sutured together. The soft palate appeared thin and tight although there was adequate movement. The hard palate was high and narrow and appeared thin and weak. The nasopharynx appeared capacious. Contact of the velum with the posterior pharyngeal wall was not observed upon phonation of /ɑ/. When the child swallowed, liquids came through the nose. She could not blow up a balloon. Sharon was referred to the cleft palate team and the voice team for evaluation.

Oral Pressure Measurements

Various types of physical measurements are used to evaluate velopharyngeal closure and oral breath pressure. A simple method is to have a child blow up a balloon with the nares open and compare this effort with that used when the nares are occluded. A carnival blower or other similar toy can be used. A spirometer can be used to measure amount of air and an oral manometer‡ to measure pressure in the oral cavity. On the oral manometer an air pressure of 8 ounces per square inch is necessary to close the nasopharynx to produce acceptable speech (97). Various types of pressure gauges§ have also been used.

Measurements on these instruments should be taken under two conditions, with the nares open and occluded. Three measurements are made for

‡ Hunter Oral Manometer, Hunter Manufacturing Company, Iowa City, Iowa 52243.

§ Emerson Resuscitator, J. H. Emerson Company, Cambridge, Massachusetts 02140.

each condition; these are averaged and a ratio between the two conditions calculated. For example, if the unoccluded reading on the oral manometer is 5 and the occluded reading is 10 (5/10), the ratio is obtained by dividing the numerator by the denominator, giving a ratio of .50. If velopharyngeal closure is achieved the readings will be the same when the nares are open as when they are occluded and the ratio would be 1.00 (10/10). The ratio may be confusing in a child with velopharyngeal insufficiency who cannot or does not increase the pressure with the nares occluded; if the child has very low pressure readings with the nares occluded and a similar low reading with the nares unoccluded the ratio would be a misleading 1.00 (82). This problem can be avoided by making sure a child exerts full effort when the nares are occluded. Morris (68) suggested conservative use of the oral manometer as an indicator of velopharyngeal competence. He felt manometer ratios are useful in predicting adequacy of velopharyngeal function for speech when used along with other test findings.

Spriestersbach, Moll, and Morris (96) established norms for this activity comparing oral manometer ratios with the mean percentage of correct consonants on an articulation test.

Manometer Ratio	Mean Percentage of Correct Consonants
.90 or more	81.40
.51 to .89	61.00
.50 or less	57.91

Other studies have also shown a positive relationship between manometer ratios and articulation skill. Pitzner and Morris (79) studied children who had cleft palates. Those who had adequate manometer ratios had articulation skills comparable to normal children. However, children with inadequate ratios had poor articulation skills on plosives, fricatives, affricates, vocalic /r/, and /l/. Barnes and Morris (5) found performance on the oral manometer was a good predictor of articulation skills.

Bernstein (9) used the oral manometer to determine manometer ratios before and after pharyngeal flap operations in patients with velopharyngeal incompetence. He found only 6% of the patients had a manometer ratio of .90 or greater before the operation but after the operation they reached this ratio in 86% of the cases.

A few cautions about the use of certain types of measures for assessing velopharyngeal competency are in order. Van Riper (102, p. 428) noted the inadequacy of testing velopharyngeal competency by ability to suck liquids up a straw, various blowing exercises, or visually observing uvular movement. Studies indicate little if any relationship of nonspeech blowing activities to velopharyngeal closure during speech. Calnan and Renfrew (23) compared x-rays of velopharyngeal closure when blowing on a carnival blower with x-rays of velopharyngeal closure during the production of the sound /i/. They concluded during blowing certain compensating muscular mechanisms were used that either did not occur or were ineffectual during the production of /i/. Prins and Bloomer (80) in studying 10 children with velopharyngeal insufficiency concluded pressure gauge readings taken during blowing activity appeared unrelated to speech intelligibility or nasality. Moll (64) as a result of cinefluorographic investigation of 10 normal subjects and 5 subjects with cleft palate, concluded ability to suck liquid through a straw or to puff the cheeks does not reflect ability to achieve velopharyngeal closure because both of these tasks can be done with only tongue-palate valving.

Air flow has been measured in evaluating velopharyngeal competence during speech. For example, Hixon, Saxman, and McQueen (41) described a technique which could be used for the clinical evaluation of velopharyngeal competence. A person wears a face mask divided into oral and nasal sections so that transmission of air between the two is impossible. The speaker may be asked to repeat /tʌ/, /kʌ/, /sʌ/, /ʃʌ/, and /fʌ/, count from 1 to 10, repeat sentences, or use connected speech under three speaking conditions, soft, normal, and loud. The amount of air emitted orally and nasally is fed separately into a device to measure the amount of nasal and oral air flow.

Velopharyngeal competency should be evaluated as objectively as possible. The conservative use of spirometer ¶ or oral pressure measures is suggested as part of the battery of tests and examinations for velopharyngeal insufficiency.

Tests for Hyponasality

Hyponasal speech, in contrast to hypernasal speech, shows an absence of nasal resonance on the /m/, /n/, and /ŋ/ sounds. Other consonants remain undisturbed but there may be slight alterations in the vowels because the normal nasal transients before and after nasal sounds are not present (also called assimilation nasality) (3, p. 685).

The examination of hyponasality should include sentences that have many /m/, /n/, and /ŋ/ sounds, such as "Mama made some lemon jam" (12). When there is definite hyponasality present the /m/ may sound like a /b/, the /n/ like a /d/, and the /ŋ/ like a /g/. The pairs of words used in testing for hypernasality can be used here (bake/make, rib/rim, dine/nine, mad/man, wig/wing, bag/bang) (94). The sound substitutions, however, would be reversed. For example, the bake/make pair would be produced

---

¶ Propper Dry Spirometer and Hutchinson Wet Spirometer, C. H. Stoelting Company, Chicago, Illinois 60624.

Name_____ Birth Date_____ Age_____ Sex_____

Rater_____ Time of Day_____ Date_____

Length of Observation_____ Place Observed_____

		Amount			Degree		
1. SHOUTING	0	1	2	3	1	2	3
2. SCREAMING	0	1	2	3	1	2	3
3. CHEERING	0	1	2	3	1	2	3
4. EXCESSIVE TALKING	0	1	2	3	1	2	3
5. STRAINED VOCALIZATIONS	0	1	2	3	1	2	3
6. REVERSE PHONATION	0	1	2	3	1	2	3
7. EXPLOSIVE RELEASE OF VOCALIZA- TIONS	0	1	2	3	1	2	3
8. ABRUPT GLOTTAL ATTACK	0	1	2	3	1	2	3
9. THROAT CLEARING	0	1	2	3	1	2	3
10. COUGHING	0	1	2	3	1	2	3
11. TALKING IN NOISE OTHER:	0	1	2	3	1	2	3

Circle appropriate numbers.

Key: Amount: 0 = None 1 = little 2 = frequent 3 = excessive

Degree: 1 = mild 2 = moderate 3 = severe

FIG. 21. Vocal abuse.

bake/bake. Hyponasality remains constant whether or not the nares are occluded.

The Identification and Analysis of Vocal Abuse

Vocal abuse must be identified and analyzed carefully. It is identified through the use of a special rating scale and analyzed by special testing.

Vocal Abuse Rating Scale

The vocal abuse rating scale (Fig. 21) contains various kinds of vocal abuses with a rating of the amount and degree of each. The rating scale includes eleven of the most common types of vocal abuses. The child should be observed in many different situations in order to assure a complete inventory of vocal abuses. These situations should include the classroom, the structured group play observation, gym, outdoor playground, and an interview with the speech clinician. Parents can be instructed in the use of the vocal abuse rating scale and asked to rate the child during various activities at home, when playing outdoors, and in other after school activities. Talking in noise should be especially noted and rated.

The *0* for none is circled if the vocal abuse is not observed, and no other rating is then made for this item. If an abuse is observed the amount and degree of each one should be carefully rated. The observed amount of each vocal abuse is indicated on a three point scale as follows: *1* little used, *2* frequently used, or *3* excessively used. The degree of severity of each vocal abuse is also rated on a three point scale: *1* mild, *2* moderate, or *3* severe. Let us look at coughing as an example. A child may cough very seldom (rating *1* in amount), but he does it in a very loud and strained manner to a severe degree (rating *3* in degree). Another child may cough very frequently (rating *3* in amount) but he does it in a mild degree (rating *1* in degree). Thus it can be seen that all combinations of amount and degree ratings are possible.

Analysis of Vocal Abuse

Vocal abuse must be analyzed carefully in a child with laryngeal dysfunction. This is done by evaluating muscular tensions during the use of a vocal abuse. Tension may appear in various muscles of the larynx, the pharynx, and the neck. Excess tension not only in the laryngeal area but in almost any area of the body may affect the voice. Van Riper (102, p. 161) stated, "Tension in any area of the body tends to flow toward and focus in the larynx." According to Isshiki and von Leden (48) vocal nodules, laryngeal edema, and other problems causing an incomplete approximation of the vocal cords cause a person to attempt to overcome this imperfect closure by contracting the laryngeal muscles with greater force; this continued forceful contraction starts a ". . . vicious circle of laryngeal hyperfunction" which is a contributing factor in voice disorders. This problem is represented by the following child.

Joyce, a 13-year-old girl, was referred by her teacher to the school speech clinician. She had a hoarse voice rated *7* on a seven point scale. She talked with great effort, taking excessively deep breaths with a raising of the shoulders. When she talked she strained so hard to phonate her face reddened and the muscles in her neck stood out, reflecting the amount of hyperfunction in the neck and shoulder areas. The laryngeal examination revealed bilateral vocal nodules at the junction of the anterior and middle thirds of the vocal cords. The nodules were approximately 2 mm. Complete approximation of the cords was hampered by the large nodules thus accounting for the extreme effort required for talking. The nodules appeared newly formed and voice therapy was recommended.

The speech clinician should determine whether the external laryngeal muscles or swallowing muscles are used in phonation. Zerffi (121–123) recommended using Kenyon's (51) finger palpation technique as the testing method. This is done by placing a finger above the larynx at the angle of the chin and asking the person to swallow. The upward movement of the larynx and muscle contractions reveal the normal cooperation of the external laryngeal muscles. Then still keeping the finger in place ask the person to speak or sing. If there are any muscular movements or upward movement of the larynx like those noted during swallowing it reveals an unnecessary involvement of the external laryngeal muscles. This indicates the vocal cords are being brought together with greater force than their muscles can tolerate causing irritation of the free edges of the vocal cords. This results in a weakening of the vocal muscles.

Indications for Voice Therapy

After all recommended diagnostic examinations including medical, psychological, audiological, and voice are completed, decisions can be made regarding rehabilitation procedures for the child. These decisions may be made in a formal type of team staffing as described under Stage II of the voice team or they may take place as a less formal type of consultation between the specialists involved.

Voice therapy may be indicated for a child either as a procedure of choice or in coordination with other forms of treatment. It is the procedure of choice under the following circumstances: (1) to determine if a laryngeal pathology can be alleviated through voice therapy prior to consideration of other treatment, (2) for adaptation to congenital or acquired anomalies, or (3) for nonorganic cases. Voice therapy is used in coordination with other treatment: (1) preceding an operation or prosthesis, (2) following an operation or prosthesis, or (3) in combination with other treatment such as medication or psychotherapy (113; 114). These indications may be followed individually or in various combinations.

Voice Therapy as the Procedure of Choice

Alleviation of Laryngeal Pathology

Voice therapy may be indicated to determine if a vocal pathology can be alleviated before other methods of treatment are considered. Laryngeal pathologies likely to respond favorably to voice therapy include vocal nodules, vocal fold thickening, diffuse polypoid conditions, hyperkeratosis, and chronic nonspecific laryngitis. This is especially true in cases where vocal misuse and vocal abuse are felt to be the cause of the laryngeal pathology. Most children with continued hoarseness due to chronic laryngitis because of vocal abuse respond favorably to improvement in speech habits (72).

Voice therapy is the treatment of choice for children with simple vocal nodules (2; 18, p. 81), particularly if the nodules seem to be soft, quite newly formed, and not fibrotic. Levbarg (53) suggested voice therapy as the treatment of choice for vocal nodules to improve the muscular tonus of the vocal cords. Brodnitz (18, p. 81) stated vocal nodules in children should not be touched as they are reversible lesions which respond well to voice therapy. Withers and Dawson (116) recommended voice therapy as the treatment of choice in certain vocal nodule cases and other times following surgical removal of the nodules. Brief voice rest followed by voice therapy may be suggested (42; 53). However, Brodnitz and Froeschels (19) stated inactivity is diametrically opposed to good principles of modern rehabilitation and there is danger of muscular atrophy because of the inactivity during voice rest. Peacher (77, p. 16) stated voice rest is not indicated in the treatment of vocal nodules but vocal education should commence immediately upon diagnosis. Peacher recognized a reduction in the amount of speaking for a time may be necessary.

Voice therapy to determine if a pathology can be alleviated must be given a good trial. Often after this trial period laryngeal conditions caused by vocal misuse and vocal abuse are definitely reduced if not absent. Even very young children can be taught to handle their voices with care and avoid flagrant vocal abuse if they are given various types of exercises appropriate for their age and interests (111).

Adaptation to Anomalies

Voice therapy may be indicated to improve a child's voice in the presence of congenital or acquired anomalies. According to Moore (65, p. 690), if the vocal mechanism is permanently altered in some way there are three compensatory objectives: (1) obtain the greatest possible use of the remaining structures; (2) develop physiological compensations; (3) help the child and his parents adjust to the different voice. Anomalies include velopharyngeal insufficiency in the absence or presence of an overt cleft palate, vocal palsy, partial paralysis of one or both vocal cords, ventricular dysphonia, and stenosis of either the pharyngeal area, the glottis, or of both. Anomalies may also be present following various types of laryngeal operations, for example scarring of the edges of the vocal cords following removal of nodules, cysts, polyps, papillomas, or laryngeal webs. Laryngeal injury may result from intubation during an operation. A few children have voice problems due to structural anomalies as a result of accidental injury to the larynx.

In marginal cases of velopharyngeal insufficiency, preliminary voice therapy sessions are indicated to see if the undesirable voice and speech habits can be eliminated. Children with velopharyngeal insufficiency who show inconsistent results on speech examinations are good candidates for voice therapy as the primary treatment. The inconsistencies may be the result of fluctuating palatopharyngeal closure associated with neuromuscular dysfunction (76) or they may be related to marginal velopharyngeal competency (69). In marginal competency a speaker may produce a good plosive but nasalize a fricative, or he may produce an acceptable pressure consonant in isolation but not in connected speech (69). In either condition the child may respond well to voice therapy. Voice therapy should be initiated if nasality persists following an operation for removal of the adenoid (8; 107). However, a child with a marked velopharyngeal incompetency will not respond favorably to voice therapy without surgical intervention or a prosthesis.

Nonorganic Problems

Voice therapy may be the preferred procedure for nonorganic problems, that is when nothing can be found wrong with the child physically. For example excessive nasality or a mutational voice problem may be seen in the absence of positive medical findings or anomalous conditions. Voice problems due to imitation are included here. Our goal under this indication is to teach new vocal habits to improve voice.

Voice Therapy in Coordination with Other Treatment

Preceding an Operation or Prosthesis

Voice therapy should begin preceding an operation (18, p. 82). For example when vocal nodules are long standing and appear hard and fibrotic an operation may be necessary. The child should be given several sessions of voice therapy before the operation for the purpose of introducing him to the principles of good voice use. This paves the way for continuation of voice therapy following the operation. For these same reasons voice therapy is sometimes recommended in cases of velopharyngeal insufficiency preceding an operation or the insertion of a prosthesis. Owsley *et al.* (76) pointed out speech improvement following surgical correction of velopharyngeal incompetence is more rapid in children who have had some preoperative speech therapy.

Following an Operation or Prosthesis

If surgical and medical procedures can provide normal or near normal structures, the speech clinician can attempt to establish adequate voice production (65, p. 690). Training in good use of voice following surgical procedures is usually necessary (53) to restore normal voice by breaking down acquired bad habits (100), to avoid a recurrence of the condition (24, p. 16), and to assure proper use of the voice (56). This is especially true when vocal misuse and vocal abuse are thought to have caused the original pathological condition (14; 67). Arnold (2) felt nodules will return after being removed if vocal abuse and vocal misuse are continued. Holinger, Johnston, and McMahon (42) stated surgical removal of small nodules may be postponed because they tend to disappear during puberty when the larynx increases in size and the stresses and strains of phonation change with the new pitch. However, if the vocal nodules do not resolve and are removed voice therapy is of great benefit following the operation. Voice training should also follow surgical removal of some hematomas and thickened vocal cord tissues (67), polyps, and polypoid thickening.

The laryngologist decides when a patient is ready for vocal rehabilitation after an operation. Some laryngologists recommend a period of voice rest others do not. Brodnitz (18, pp. 82–84) suggested voice rest during healing with no whispering for a few days up to longer periods. He stated the periods of voice rest vary according to pathology. Vocal nodules and small pedunculated polyps require a few days to a week, sessile polyps require about 2 weeks, and larger polypoid thickenings may require a longer period. He recommended voice therapy should be initiated immediately after voice rest. Loré (57, p. 392) stated following vocal cord stripping, the procedure he prefers for most lesions involving the vocal cords, the patient should be allowed to talk immediately after the operation but with certain restrictions. He should not be allowed to talk excessively, whisper, shout, or sing for a period of 3 to 5 weeks.

In a few cases postoperative voice therapy may be indicated because the the child clings unnecessarily to his defective manner of speaking. A hoarse voice may persist after successful surgical procedures because it sounds natural to the child.

In cases of velopharyngeal insufficiency voice therapy is indicated following surgical procedures (37) or insertion of a prosthetic speech aid. Berner (8) also suggested if good speech is not regained following adenotonsillectomy it may be necessary to consider palate lengthening, pharyngeal flap, or pharyngoplasty; these surgical procedures may be performed alone or in combination. Voice therapy may be recommended following such procedures.

In Combination with Other Treatment

Sometimes voice therapy is conducted concurrently with other treatment such as psychological-psychiatric, medical, and physical therapy.

Psychological-Psychiatric. Emphasis should be placed on psychological factors as well as physiological factors in a person with a vocal disturbance (18, p. 80; 67). Many patients with voice problems need psychiatric consultation and treatment, some need only guidance and the solution of minor problems, but others need psychiatric referral (1; 54). A psychological approach freeing the patient of problems through sympathetic understanding may be necessary (16). Vocal rehabilitation should not be based only upon the condition of the larynx but the speech clinician must also have an understanding of the personality of the client (11). Psychiatric help may be indicated in cases of vocal nodules when excitement, worry, fear, and anxiety are detrimental to good voice use (53). Psychotherapy is indicated in some cases of infantile personality where there has been a continuation of high pitch levels into and through adolescence (102, p. 160). Psychotherapy should be part of the treatment of incomplete mutation because of the frequent accompanying emotional disturbances (58, p. 194). Psychotherapy may be an adjunct to voice therapy in ventricular phonation (58, p. 320). Psychotherapeutic measures may be indicated if a child needs better adjustment and a less aggressive personality (2; 58, p. 184).

People with laryngeal dysfunction are apt to be gregarious, talkative, and physically active (67). Vocal nodules will often recur after removal in the overly active shouting boy if his personality remains unchanged (42). Hysterical dysphonia or aphonia in adolescence is of concern to the laryngologist, the psychiatrist or psychologist, and the speech clinician. A child with long standing hysterical aphonia may need direction and instruction in good voice production. For example, Wolski and Wiley (117) reported the successful treatment of functional aphonia in a 14-year-old boy who had become aphonic 6 months previously following laryngitis. Voice therapy was coordinated with psychiatric treatment with a normal voice the result.

Medical. Many children with laryngeal dysfunction are overly active. The physician may recommend placing a child on medication during voice therapy. We have seen such children become much more vocally manageable when receiving proper medication. Medication in some cases produces a favorable atmosphere and relaxation of physical tensions; tranquilizers may be indicated, hormonal treatment may be used in metabolic deficiencies, and corticosteroids may reduce allergic conditions (16). Hormonal treatment may be indicated in cases of incomplete voice mutation where slight endocrine deficiences are found (58, p. 194).

Physical Therapy. In cases of ventricular phonation, physical therapy including heat and vibratory massage of the neck along with voice therapy is sometimes suggested (58, p. 320). In the hands of a physician or properly qualified person a weak electric current may relax muscles for better production of voice while a stronger current may stimulate muscular activity if stimulation is necessary for better voice (16). Shelton (90) in discussing therapeutic exercise and speech pathology concluded ". . . the speech clinician should concentrate on the development of speech skill and leave remediation of the speech mechanism to physicians." The coordination of both aspects may result in facilitating voice improvement.

Prognosis in Voice Disorders

Prognosis, the prediction of the outcome of voice therapy, depends upon the individual child and his particular problem. A prognosis is based upon the cause of the problem, examination results, indications for therapy, and the planned therapy procedures. We recognize a prognosis for an individual child cannot be made until the treatment plan has been formulated. However, we feel the speech clinician should keep a tentative prognosis in mind while formulating therapy plans. Therefore, we are discussing prognosis before presenting material the speech clinician will use in making specific plans for therapy.

A prognosis may be favorable, unfavorable, or guarded. A favorable prognosis indicates that a child upon completion of his therapy program will have a much improved or corrected voice. An unfavorable prognosis means the opposite, that is the outlook is negative regarding the end result of voice therapy. A guarded prognosis indicates a question about improvement in voice for many reasons including cooperation of child and parents, associated physical or psychological problems, or the very nature of the voice problem itself.

Success in improving voice rests squarely on the client's desire for improvement (78, p. 863). Motivation to improve voice is a special problem with children. Motivation must be stimulated to a high degree; we must carefully assess the degree of motivation in a child to improve his voice; progress with some children who state they want to change their voice habits may be slow because of unconscious resistance to therapy (104, pp. 274–275). Motivation is not too difficult if we plan a therapy program carefully and then present it to the child in clear cut step-by-step fashion so he knows what is wrong with his voice and what is going to be done to help him improve it.

A favorable prognosis for therapy is indicated if we can get a better voice from a child under maximum clinical stimulation in a brief teaching period (100). Van Riper and Dopheide (103) recommended the inclusion of a trial period of therapy during diagnostic evaluations. They stated even a 20-min period may reveal much about a person's motivation, cooperation, and difficulties. The ability to produce a clear voice upon stimulation does not mean the problem will resolve itself without training; rather it means voice therapy has a good chance of being successful. Thus a child who can produce a better voice under clinical stimulation should not be eliminated from voice therapy (106).

Prognosis depends to a large degree upon the amount of therapy time available. It is more favorable if a child can be seen on a regular basis. If possible a child should be seen daily during the first week or two. After this the sessions should be scheduled so he is seen for 20 to 40 hourly sessions of voice therapy during a 12-week period to see if the pathology can be alleviated. Frequent brief periods of practice are often recommended. For laryngeal dysfunction Peacher (77, p. 10) recommended 2- to 5-min practice sessions about 20 times a day for the initial week or two of therapy. Moore (65, p. 695) suggested frequent short practice sessions avoiding overuse of the voice. He recommended only 3 min an hour gradually increasing the length of practice sessions until an occasional practice session of 30 min might be attempted. During the 12-week period the child may be rechecked by the laryngologist or seen by other members of the voice team. The total voice therapy time is usually 4 or 5 months in cases of vocal nodules (77, p. 16).

Prognosis for laryngeal dysfunction depends upon many factors and in most cases is favorable. Van Riper and Irwin (104, p. 189) stated, "Prognosis in voice cases where vocal nodules are present depends upon the location and size of the nodules, their duration, and the necessity for surgery, and the case's ability to change his habits of phonation." When hoarseness is a result of excessive use of the voice, improvement will be proportionate to the success in correcting the vocal abuse (75). The prognosis for children with vocal nodules depends upon controlling vocal abuse and helping the child develop a less aggressive pattern of vocal expression through voice therapy (58, p. 186). Vocal nodules should show a reduction in size within 3 months of voice therapy (109, p. 218). Children with hoarseness because of chronic laryngitis occasionally require prolonged voice therapy (72). Inflammation due to hyperkinetic dysphonia is usually decreased after a month's therapy (38, p. 121). Saunders (86) stated the prognosis in dysphonia plicae ventricularis usually should be guarded as some patients remain hoarse despite all efforts to help them. However, Luchsinger (58, p. 32) stated generally the prognosis is quite favorable in ventricular phonation unless there is a serious neurosis present.

Prognosis can be exemplified by Baynes' (7) program. Fourteen children with vocal nodules and vocal cord thickening had small group therapy 2 hours a week for a period of 8 weeks. The children were reexamined by a laryngologist 12 weeks after the initiation of the program. Seven of the children exhibited normal vocal cords without any pathology remaining. Four of the children showed a definite decrease in the amount of vocal cord thickening and three of the children did not continue in the program throughout this period. It was found as voice quality improved pathology diminished.

If the aim is to adjust to structural anomalies, in most cases the prognosis must be quite guarded (109, p. 216). This is especially true with anomalies of the laryngeal area and with velopharyngeal insufficiency. These conditions may require extensive therapy often lasting many months. In cases of velopharyngeal insufficiency Barnes and Morris (5) suggested the speech clinician should recheck sounds incorrectly produced on the articulation test to see if the child can produce the sounds correctly after stimulation. If so this indicates a potential for good velopharyngeal competence and gives a favorable prognosis.

In nonorganic cases the prognosis must be guarded since it depends in part upon unknown factors. Overall exposure time to voice therapy varies. The prognosis varies according to the child and the presenting problem in children with functional voice problems. These problems include hypernasality in the absence of structural deviations, problems of hoarseness with no organic basis, pitch deviations, and problems of loudness. The prognosis for persistent falsetto in the young male is especially favorable (58, p. 197; 108).

When voice therapy is coordinated or combined with other treatment the prognosis is dependent to a large extent on the prognosis for the other treatment. In cases in which an operation or prosthesis is necessary the prognosis is always better if the child is given several sessions of voice therapy before these procedures. Brodnitz (14) recommended beginning with 2 or 3 sessions a week following removal of cord lesions with the average length of voice therapy about 2 months. Progress in psychotherapy may determine progress in voice therapy. Medication may relieve physical conditions contributing to the voice problem. Physical therapy may improve the balance of muscular tonus. Progress in other therapies speeds progress in voice and improves the voice prognosis.

We have discussed the type and extent of examination procedures necessary for a child with a voice problem. Selecting the examinations for a particular child depends upon the presenting voice problem and associated problems. The physical examinations and a case history concentrating on the child's problems are basic to all examination procedures. Examinations are carefully selected and administered by the speech clinician. In formulating therapy plans the indications for therapy and a tentative prognosis are kept in mind.

REFERENCES

1. Alfaro, V. R. Psychogenic influences in otolaryngology. *Arch. Otolaryng. (Chicago)*, **71**, 1960, 11–17.
2. Arnold, G. E. Vocal nodules and polyps: Laryngeal tissue reaction to habitual hyperkinetic dysphonia. *J. Speech Hearing Dis.*, **27**, 1962, 205–216.
3. Arnold, G. E. Physiology and pathology of speech and language. In R. Luchsinger and G. E. Arnold. *Voice—speech—language. Clinical communicology: Its physiology and pathology.* Belmont: Wadsworth Publishing Company, 1965.
4. Arnold, G. E. Advances in laryngeal physiology and their clinical application. *Eye, Ear, Nose, Throat Monthly*, **45**, 1966, 78–84.
5. Barnes, I. J., and Morris, H. L. Interrelationships among oral breath pressure ratios and articulation skills for individuals with cleft palate. *J. Speech Hearing Res.*, **10**, 1967, 506–514.
6. Baynes, R. A. Clinical observations of children with voice disorders. *J. Michigan Speech Hearing Ass.*, **1**, 1965, 10–12.
7. Baynes, R. A. Voice therapy with children: A global approach. *J. Michigan Speech Hearing Ass.*, **3**, 1967, 11–14.
8. Berner, R. E. Hazards of adenotonsillectomy in the child with cleft palate. *JAMA*, **181**, 1962, 558–559.
9. Bernstein, L. Treatment of velopharyngeal incompetence. *Arch. Otolaryng. (Chicago)*, **85**, 1967, 67–74.
10. Black, J. W. Relationships among fundamental frequency, vocal sound pressure, and rate of speaking. *Lang. Speech*, **4**, 1961, 196–199.
11. Bloch, P. New limits of vocal analysis. *Folia Phoniat. (Basel)*, **12**, 1960, 291–297.

12. Bloomer, H. H., and Wolski, W. Office examination of palatopharyngeal function. *Clin. Pediat. (Phila.)*, **7**, 1968, 611–618.
13. Bradford, L. J., Brooks, A. R., and Shelton, R. L., Jr. Clinical judgment of hypernasality in cleft palate children. *Cleft Palate J.*, **1**, 1964, 329–335.
14. Brodnitz, F. S. Post-operative vocal rehabilitation in benign lesions of the vocal cord. *Folia Phoniat. (Basel)*, **7**, 1955, 193–200.
15. Brodnitz, F. S. The pressure test in mutational voice disturbances. *Ann. Otol.*, **67**, 1958, 235–240.
16. Brodnitz, F. S. Vocal rehabilitation in benign lesions of the vocal cords. *J. Speech Hearing Dis.*, **23**, 1958, 112–117.
17. Brodnitz, F. S. The holistic study of the voice. *Quart. J. Speech*, **48**, 1962, 280–284.
18. Brodnitz, F. S. *Vocal rehabilitation.* Ed. 3. Rochester, Minn.: American Academy of Ophthalmology and Otolaryngology, 1965.
19. Brodnitz, F. S., and Froeschels, E. Treatment of vocal nodules by chewing method. *Arch. Otolaryng. (Chicago)*, **59**, 1954, 560–565.
20. Brookshire, R. H. Speech pathology and the experimental analysis of behavior. *J. Speech Hearing Dis.*, **32**, 1967, 215–227.
21. Buck, M. Post-operative velo-pharyngeal movements in cleft palate cases. *J. Speech Hearing Dis.*, **19**, 1954, 288–294.
22. Calnan, J. Submucous cleft palate. *Brit. J. Plast. Surg.*, **6**, 1954, 264–282.
23. Calnan, J., and Renfrew, C. E. Blowing tests and speech. *Brit. J. Plast. Surg.*, **13**, 1961, 340–346.
24. Clerf, L. H. Laryngeal disease and voice therapy. In *Proceedings of the first institute on voice pathology, and the first international meeting of laryngectomized persons.* Cleveland Hearing and Speech Center, 1952.
25. Collins, E. G. *A guide to diseases of the nose, throat and ear for general practitioners and students.* Baltimore: Williams and Wilkins Company, 1964.
26. Cullinan, W. L., and Counihan, D. T. Some factors affecting the size of Q values for speech ratings. *Percept. Motor Skills*, **27**, 1968, 531–536.
27. Curry, E. T. The pitch characteristics of the adolescent male voice. *Speech Monogr.*, **7**, 1940, 48–62.
28. Curtis, J. F. Disorders of voice. In W. Johnson and D. Moeller (Editors). *Speech handicapped school children.* Ed. 3. New York: Harper and Row, 1967.
29. DeWeese, D. D., and Saunders, W. H. *Textbook of otolaryngology.* Ed. 3. St. Louis: C. V. Mosby Company, 1968.
30. Duffy, R. J. Fundamental frequency characteristics of adolescent females. *Lang. Speech*, **13**, 1970, 14–24.
31. Fairbanks, G. *Voice and articulation drillbook.* Ed. 2. New York: Harper and Brothers, 1960.
32. Fairbanks, G., Herbert, E. L., and Hammond, J. M. An acoustical study of vocal pitch in seven- and eight-year-old girls. *Child Develop.*, **20**, 1949, 71–78.
33. Fairbanks, G., Wiley, J. H., and Lassman, F. M. An acoustical study of vocal pitch in seven- and eight-year-old boys. *Child Develop.*, **20**, 1949, 63–69.
34. Fletcher, H. *Speech and hearing in communication.* Princeton: D. Van Nostrand Company, 1953.
35. Freeman, G. G. County speech services: A clinical program in the public schools. *Asha*, **3**, 1961, 46–47.
36. Freeman, G. G. Innovative school programs: The Oakland schools plan. *J. Speech Hearing Dis.*, **34**, 1969, 220–225.
37. Goda, S. Speech therapy with selected patients with congenital velopharyngeal inadequacy. *Cleft Palate J.*, **3**, 1966, 268–274.
38. Greene, M. C. L. *The voice and its disorders.* Ed. 2. Philadelphia: J. B. Lippincott Company, 1964.
39. Gutzmann, H. Diagnostik und therapie der funktionellen stimmstoerungen. *Med.-Paedagog. Monatsschr. f. d. ges. Sprachheilkunde*, **20**, 1910, 55. Cited by Brodnitz, F. S. The pressure test in mutational voice disturbances. *Ann. Otol.*, **67**, 1958, 235–240.

98 VOICE PROBLEMS OF CHILDREN

40. Hagerty, R., and Hoffmeister, F. S. Velopharyngeal closure; an index of speech. *J. Plast. Reconstr. Surg.*, **13**, 1954, 290–298.
41. Hixon, T. J., Saxman, J. H., and McQueen, H. D. The respirometric technique for evaluating velopharyngeal competence during speech. *Folia Phoniat. (Basel)*, **19**, 1967, 203–219.
42. Holinger, P., Johnston, K. C., and McMahon, R. J. Hoarseness in infants and children. *Eye, Ear, Nose, Throat Monthly*, **31**, 1952, 247–251.
43. Hollien, H., and Malcik, E. Adolescent voice change in southern Negro males. *Speech Monogr.*, **29**, 1962, 53–58.
44. Hollien, H., and Malcik, E. Evaluation of cross-sectional studies of adolescent voice change in males. *Speech Monogr.*, **34**, 1967, 80–84.
45. Hollien, H., Malcik, E., and Hollien, B. Adolescent voice change in southern white males. *Speech Monogr.*, **32**, 1965, 87–90.
46. Hollien, H., and Paul, P. A second evaluation of the speaking fundamental frequency characteristics of post-adolescent girls. *Lang. Speech*, **12**, 1969, 119–124.
47. Irwin, R. B. *Speech and hearing therapy. Clinical and educational principles and practices*. Pittsburgh: Stanwix House, 1965.
48. Isshiki, N., and von Leden, H. Hoarseness: Aerodynamic studies. *Arch. Otolaryng. (Chicago)*, **80**, 1964, 206–213.
49. Johnson, W., Darley, F. L., and Spriestersbach, D. C. *Diagnostic methods in speech pathology*. New York: Harper and Row, 1963.
50. Kaplan, E. N., Jobe, R. P., and Chase, R. A. Flexibility in surgical planning for velopharyngeal incompetence. *Cleft Palate J.*, **6**, 1969, 166–174.
51. Kenyon, E. L. Action and control of peripheral organs of speech: Psychologic principles, and scientific basis for methods of training. *JAMA*, **91**, 1928, 1341–1346.
52. Launer, P. G. Maximum phonation time in children. Unpublished master's thesis, State University of New York at Buffalo, 1971.
53. Levbarg, J. J. Vocal therapy *versus* surgery for the eradication of singers' and speakers' nodules. *Eye, Ear, Nose, Throat Monthly*, **18**, 1939, 81–82, 91.
54. Lewy, R. B. Practical aspects of psychiatry applied to otolaryngology. *Arch. Otolaryng., (Chicago)*, **77**, 1963, 444–446.
55. Lintz, L. B., and Sherman, D. Phonetic elements and perception of nasality. *J. Speech Hearing Res.*, **4**, 1961, 381–396.
56. Loré, J. M., Jr. Hoarseness in children. *Arch. Otolaryng. (Chicago)*, **51**, 1950, 814–825.
57. Loré, J. M., Jr. *An atlas of head and neck surgery*. Philadelphia: W. B. Saunders Company, 1962.
58. Luchsinger, R. Physiology and pathology of respiration and phonation. In R. Luchsinger and G. E. Arnold. *Voice—speech—language. Clinical communicology: Its physiology and pathology*. Belmont: Wadsworth Publishing Company, 1965.
59. McGlone, R. E. Vocal pitch characteristics of children aged one to two years. *Speech Monogr.*, **33**, 1966, 178–181.
60. Massengill, R., Jr. An objective technique for submucous cleft palate detection. *J. Plast. Reconstr. Surg.*, **37**, 1966, 355–359.
61. Michel, J. F., Hollien, H., and Moore, P. Speaking fundamental frequency characteristics of 15-, 16-, and 17-year-old girls. *Lang. Speech*, **9**, 1965, 46–51.
62. Milisen, R. Methods of evaluation and diagnosis of speech disorders. In L. E Travis (Editor). *Handbook of speech pathology*. New York: Appleton-Century-Crofts, Inc., 1957.
63. Moll, K. L. Velopharyngeal closure on vowels. *J. Speech Hearing Res.*, **5**, 1962, 30–37.
64. Moll, K. L. A cinefluorographic study of velopharyngeal function in normals during various activities. *Cleft Palate J.*, **2**, 1965, 112–122.
65. Moore, G. P. Voice disorders associated with organic abnormalities. In L. E.

Travis (Editor). *Handbook of speech pathology*. New York: Appleton-Century-Crofts, Inc., 1957.
66. Moore, M. V. Help for the child with a voice disorder. *Alabama School J.*, **84,** 1967, 30–31, 40, 42.
67. Moore, P. Treatment of voice defects following surgery. *Conn. Med. J.*, **19,** 1955, 180–183.
68. Morris, H. L. The oral manometer as a diagnostic tool in clinical speech pathology. *J. Speech Hearing Dis.*, **31,** 1966, 362–369.
69. Morris, H. L., and Smith, J. K. A multiple approach for evaluating velopharyngeal competency. *J. Speech Hearing Dis.*, **27,** 1962, 218–226.
70. Morris, H. L., Spriestersbach, D. C., and Darley, F. L. An articulation test for assessing competency of velopharyngeal closure. *J. Speech Hearing Res.*, **4,** 1961, 48–55.
71. Murphy, A. T. *Functional voice disorders*. Englewood Cliffs: Prentice-Hall, Inc., 1964.
72. Murphy, R. S. Hoarseness. *Nova Scotia Med. Bull.*, **46,** 1967, 177–179.
73. Myklebust, H. R. *Development and disorders of written language. Volume One. Picture story language test*. New York: Grune and Stratton, 1965.
74. O'Neill, J. J., and McGee, J. A. Management of benign laryngeal tumors in children: Preoperative, operative and postoperative. *Ann. Otol.*, **71,** 1962, 480–488.
75. Orton, H. B. The significance of hoarseness. *New Orleans Med. Surg. J.*, **103,** 1951, 511–515.
76. Owsley, J. Q., Jr., Chierici, G., Miller, E. R., Lawson, L. I., and Blackfield, H. M. Cephalometric evaluation of palatal dysfunction in patients without cleft palate. *J. Plast. Reconstr. Surg.*, **39,** 1967, 562–568.
77. Peacher, G. Voice therapy for ulcers and nodules of the larynx. In *Proceedings of the first institute on voice pathology, and the first international meeting of laryngectomized persons*. Cleveland Hearing and Speech Center, 1952.
78. Perkins, W. H. The challenge of functional disorders of voice. In L. E. Travis (Editor). *Handbook of speech pathology*. New York: Appleton-Century-Crofts, Inc., 1957.
79. Pitzner, J. C., and Morris, H. L. Articulation skills and adequacy of breath pressure ratios of children with cleft palate. *J. Speech Hearing Dis.*, **31,** 1966, 26–40.
80. Prins, D., and Bloomer, H. H. A word intelligibility approach to the study of speech change in oral cleft patients. *Cleft Palate J.*, **2,** 1965, 357–368.
81. Ptacek, P. H., and Sander, E. K. Maximum duration of phonation. *J. Speech Hearing Dis.*, **28,** 1963, 171–182.
82. Quigley, L. F., Jr. Pressure and cephalometric technics for evaluation of normal and cleft palate patients. II. Palatopharyngeal competency. *J. Dent. Res.*, **47,** 1968, 760–768.
83. Rees, M. Some variables affecting perceived harshness. *J. Speech Hearing Res.*, **1,** 1958, 155–168.
84. Rise, E. N. Velopharyngeal incompetence. *Southern Med. J.*, **59,** 1966, 337–340.
85. Rubin, H. J. Role of the laryngologist in management of dysfunctions of the singing voice. *Trans. Pacif. Coast Otoophthal. Soc.*, **45,** 1964, 57–77.
86. Saunders, W. H. Dysphonia plicae ventricularis: An overlooked condition causing chronic hoarseness. *Ann. Otol.*, **65,** 1956, 665–673.
87. Saunders, W. H. The larynx. *Clin. Sympos.*, **16,** 1964, 67–99.
88. Sawashima, M. Measurement of phonation time. *Jap. J. Logopedics Phoniat.*, 1966, 23–28. Cited by Sawashima, M., Totsuka, G., Kobayashi, T., and Hirose, H. Surgery for hoarseness due to unilateral vocal cord paralysis. *Arch. Otolaryng. (Chicago)*, **87,** 1968, 289–294.
89. Sawashima, M., Totsuka, G., Kobayashi, T., and Hirose, H. Surgery for hoarseness due to unilateral vocal cord paralysis. *Arch. Otolaryng. (Chicago)*, **87,** 1968, 289–294.

90. Shelton, R. L., Jr. Therapeutic exercise and speech pathology. *Asha*, **5**, 1963, 855–859.
91. Shelton, R. L., Jr., Brooks, A. R., and Youngstrom, K. A. Clinical assessment of palatopharyngeal closure. *J. Speech Hearing Dis.*, **30**, 1965, 37–43.
92. Sherman, D., and Linke, E. The influence of certain vowel types on degree of harsh voice quality. *J. Speech Hearing Dis.*, **17**, 1952, 401–408.
93. Sherman, D., and Moodie, C. E. Four psychological scaling methods applied to articulation defectiveness. *J. Speech Hearing Dis.*, **22**, 1957, 698–706.
94. Shupe, L. K. Speech intelligibility measures of cleft palate speakers before and after pharyngeal flap surgery. Unpublished Ph.D. dissertation, State University of New York at Buffalo, 1968.
95. Spriestersbach, D. C. Routine methods of examination and diagnosis of velopharyngeal incompetency. Speech aspects. *Cleft Palate Bull.*, **8**, 1958, 7–8.
96. Spriestersbach, D. C., Moll, K. L., and Morris, H. L. Subject classification and articulation of speakers with cleft palate. *J. Speech Hearing Res.*, **4**, 1961, 362–372.
97. Spriestersbach, D. C., and Powers, G. R. Articulation skills, velopharyngeal closure, and oral breath pressure of children with cleft palates. *J. Speech Hearing Res.*, **2**, 1959, 318–325.
98. Subtelny, J. D., and Koepp-Baker, H. The significance of adenoid tissue in velopharyngeal function. *J. Plast. Reconstr. Surg.*, **17**, 1956, 235–250.
99. Subtelny, J. D., Koepp-Baker, H., and Subtelny, J. D. Palatal function and cleft palate speech. *J. Speech Hearing Dis.*, **26**, 1961, 213–224.
100. Tarneaud, J. The fundamental principles of vocal cultivation and therapeutics of the voice. *Logos*, **1**, 1958, 7–10.
101. Templin, M. C., and Darley, F. L. *The Templin-Darley tests of articulation—A manual and discussion of articulation testing.* Ed. 2. Iowa City: Bureau of Educational Research and Service, University of Iowa, 1969.
102. Van Riper, C. *Speech correction. Principles and methods.* Ed. 4. Englewood Cliffs: Prentice-Hall, Inc., 1963.
103. Van Riper, C., and Dopheide, W. Diagnostic services in a training center. *Asha*, **8**, 1966, 37–39.
104. Van Riper, C., and Irwin, J. V. *Voice and articulation.* Englewood Cliffs: Prentice-Hall, Inc., 1958.
105. Villarreal, J. Consistency of judgments of voice quality. *Southern Speech J.*, **15**, 1950, 10–20.
106. Webster, E. J., Perkins, W. H., Bloomer, H. H., and Pronovost, W. Case selection in the schools. *J. Speech Hearing Dis.*, **31**, 1966, 352–358.
107. Weiss, D. A. Organic lesions leading to speech disorders. *Nervous Child.*, **7**, 1948, 29–37.
108. Weiss, D. A. The pubertal change of the human voice. *Folia Phoniat. (Basel)*, **2**, 1950, 127–158.
109. West, R. W., and Ansberry, M. *The rehabilitation of speech.* Ed. 4. New York: Harper and Row, 1968.
110. Westphal, W. *Physikalisches Worterbuch.* Vienna: Springer, 1952. Cited in R. Luchsinger and G. E. Arnold. *Voice—speech—language. Clinical communicology: Its physiology and pathology.* Belmont: Wadsworth Publishing Company, 1965.
111. Wilson, D. K. Children with vocal nodules. *J. Speech Hearing Dis.*, **26**, 1961, 19–26.
112. Wilson, D. K. The hearing team. *Volta Rev.*, **64**, 1962, 22–25.
113. Wilson, D. K. Voice re-education in benign laryngeal pathology. *Eye, Ear, Nose, Throat Monthly*, **45**, 1966, 76–80.
114. Wilson, D. K. Voice therapy for children with laryngeal dysfunction. *Southern Med. J.*, **61**, 1968, 956–958.
115. Wilson, M. E. A standardized method for obtaining a spoken language sample. *J. Speech Hearing Res.*, **12**, 1969, 95–102.

116. Withers, B. R., and Dawson, M. H. Psychological aspects. Treatment of vocal nodule cases. *Texas State J. Med.*, **56**, 1960, 43–46.
117. Wolski, W., and Wiley, J. Functional aphonia in a fourteen-year-old boy: A case report. *J. Speech Hearing Dis.*, **30**, 1965, 71–75.
118. Yanagihara, N. Significance of harmonic changes and noise components in hoarseness. *J. Speech Hearing Res.*, **10**, 1967, 531–541.
119. Yanagihara, N., and Koike, Y. The regulation of sustained phonation. *Folia Phoniat. (Basel)*, **19**, 1967, 1–18.
120. Yanagihara, N., Koike, Y., and von Leden, H. Phonation and respiration. Function study in normal subjects. *Folia Phoniat. (Basel)*, **18**, 1966, 323–340.
121. Zerffi, W. A. C. Functional vocal disabilities. *Laryngoscope*, **49**, 1939, 1143–1147.
122. Zerffi, W. A. C. Voice re-education. *Arch. Otolaryng. (Chicago)*, **48**, 1948, 521–526.
123. Zerffi, W. A. C. Laryngology and voice production. *Ann. Otol.*, **61**, 1952, 642–647.

4

VOICE THERAPY—SOME BASIC
APPROACHES

We have seen that each child with a voice problem needs special appraisal and diagnostic techniques specifically designed for him. At this point we are concerned mainly with therapy procedures from an overall point of view. Later we will present procedures for specific voice problems.

During the initial part of the voice therapy program the child should be taught how voice is produced and given basic facts about his voice problem (30; 31). The level and detail of instruction are dependent upon the age and intelligence of the child. Having a basic understanding of vocal function and malfunction enables him to understand therapy procedures and serves to motivate him to improve his voice. A young child can be given a simplified explanation of how the larynx functions and how the laryngeal tone is resonated and articulated to form meaningful speech communication. The cause of his defective voice can be explained without elaborate detail. A young child responds best to drawings made by the clinician as the child's problem is discussed. For example vocal nodules can be compared to calluses on the hands or merely called "bumps" on the vocal cords. Older children and adolescents benefit not only from drawings but also from carefully selected charts from anatomy books and models (12, pp. 188–189). Care should be taken to avoid drawings that might be considered too detailed or too pathologically oriented. These explanations are particularly beneficial when the child must be given reasons for modifying or eliminating vocal abuse and vocal misuse (32).

Children are seen individually and in groups organized according to type and severity of voice problems. The basic program for improving voice includes the following: (1) listening training, (2) teaching correct voice use, (3) negative practice, and (4) habituation of new vocal patterns. Elimination or modification of vocal abuse and vocal misuse is important with many voice problems. The role of the family during all stages of vocal rehabilitation is stressed. Consideration is given to emotional and social problems of the child with a voice problem. Structured therapy using psychotherapeutic methods forms an integral part of the program. Atten-

102

tion is given to the application of operant conditioning principles and methods. Throughout a therapy program the clinician must keep detailed records of each session and write periodic progress reports.

Listening Training

A key to attaining almost all of the goals of voice therapy is the application of carefully programmed listening training procedures. The child is first taught to recognize the difference between a good voice and a poor voice (8; 12, p. 189; 22, p. 110; 28, p. 179). As the term listening training implies the child is the listener. A child is given experience identifying poor voice use while listening to the clinician's voice and sometimes to the voices of other children with voice problems (21, p. 692). Through listening to others a child learns to identify defective aspects of voice including vocal misuse and vocal abuse. The speech clinician uses the defective aspects present in the child's voice. These may be a vocal abuse, too high pitch level, overly loud voice, hoarseness, hypernasality, or hyponasality. If vocal abuses are present elimination or modification of these abuses should be approached early in therapy. Listening material should be live or prerecorded on a tape recorder, a language master, or other type of machine. All productions should be consistent from sample to sample. The three steps of listening training for a child with a voice deviation are (a) awareness of the deviation in others, (b) gross discrimination of differences in others, and (c) fine discrimination of differences in others.

Awareness of Differences in Others

In this step the child becomes aware of the defective aspect. The speech clinician demonstrates the defective aspect and points out the identifying features. The clinician then produces sounds, syllables, words, and sentences with the defective aspect on some. The child signals the occurrence of the defective aspect; for example the child indicates when the clinician's voice is hoarse. A scoring system should be devised to enable the child to tabulate his responses. Rewards for correct responses may be appropriate. Baynes (2) developed awareness of differences in children by teaching them differences between various voice qualities by listening to each other. Brief recordings were made of each child in the group. They then listened to an unidentified recording of a member of the group and were asked to identify the person from the recording. In a like manner, children were taught to distinguish loud from soft voices and high-pitched voices from low-pitched voices. Each child was immediately rewarded for correct responses by receiving a point after his name listed on a chart.

Gross Discrimination of Differences in Others

The second step in listening training is gross discrimination of differences. The speech clinician explains the identifying features of two levels of voice production, the correct and incorrect. The child is then asked only to discriminate between the two productions, using the same-different technique. That is, pairs of the speech clinician's vocal productions are judged by the child as being the same or different. Some pairs have two correct vocal productions, other pairs have one correct and one defective production, and other pairs have both defective. This can be done live or recorded. The speech clinician can record many pairs on language master cards. The child can run the cards through the language master and stack the cards in appropriate piles. Next the child identifies each adequate and each inadequate production in the pairs. He now identifies the characteristics of each production. For example he listens to pairs and identifies the first one in the pair as hoarse and the second one clear, both productions as clear, or both as hoarse.

In listening training with the same-different technique the material at first should contain more different than same pairs. It takes a longer time to determine if two identical stimuli are the same than to determine if two dissimilar stimuli are different (3). Thus a child can experience more success initially if he is asked to discriminate between pairs that are different.

Fine Discrimination of Differences in Others

The third procedure in listening training is fine discrimination of differences. At least three levels of vocal performance are selected for the child to discriminate. The differences between the levels are reduced as the child becomes more proficient, requiring him eventually to discriminate very fine differences. The three levels are demonstrated by the clinician and their identifying characteristics explained. For example the speech clinician records three vowels on a language master at different pitch levels, high, middle, and low. Other cards can be recorded with the order scrambled. For hypernasality the speech clinician uses excessive hypernasality, moderate hypernasality, and normal resonance. For hoarseness, the child is asked to discriminate between a voice that has moderate hoarseness, one with mild hoarseness, and one with no hoarseness. The child listens to the three productions and identifies each one according to the descriptions provided by the clinician. For example, for pitch identification he must tell which productions are high, middle, and low.

Listening training is most effective when a visual stimulus is presented simultaneously with an auditory stimulus (11). Karlovich (13) asked young adults to judge sensation levels of pure tones when the tones were accompanied by a light flash. He found ". . . that visual stimulation presented in synchrony with an auditory stimulus can influence the perception of the magnitude of the auditory stimulus." He found simultaneous presentation of a visual stimulus and a standard auditory stimulus caused the auditory stimulus to be perceived as louder by the subjects. We have found more effective listening training can be done when auditory stimuli are accompanied by visual stimuli. Accompanying visual stimuli for younger children can be simple drawings. For older children sounds or words can be written on language master cards to reinforce the auditory input.

Teaching Correct Voice Use

Completion of a thorough program in listening training gives the child the basis for producing an improved voice. The basic procedures for teaching improved voice parallel the listening training program. Here, however, the child becomes the performer and the speech clinician the listener. Production of correct voice follows three steps (33). (1) Awareness of the deviation in his own voice: The child is taught to recognize his own incorrect use of a specific voice parameter. (2) Gross discrimination of differences in his own voice: He is asked to produce two levels of the voice characteristic, the correct and incorrect. (3) Fine discrimination of differences in his own voice: He produces three levels of the specific voice parameter.

The problem of hoarseness can be used to illustrate these three steps. (1) To develop awareness of the deviation in his own voice the child listens to tape recordings of his own production of vowels. The clinician uses a random arrangement of hoarse and clear vowels selected from the diagnostic tests. The child signals each time he hears a hoarse vowel and is rewarded appropriately. (2) The child then progresses to the next step, gross discrimination of differences. Here he produces vowels or words containing the old hoarse quality and contrasts them with his best approximation to the desired quality. The clinician selects vowels on which the child can achieve some success for initial practice. These productions can be tape recorded on language master cards and the child can stack the cards into the piles representing his two types of production. (3) The child next proceeds to fine discrimination in his own voice using three degrees of hoarseness, his old faulty hoarse voice, an intermediate amount of hoarseness, and his closest approximation to clear voice. These, too, may be recorded on tape or language master cards. If the child experiences difficulty producing intermediate stages of this defective quality, the clinician may prefer not to have the child spend much time on discrimination of fine differences in his own voice. It may be more productive to spend time teaching the child correct production rather than an intermediate stage. However, using several levels of quality in his own voice may serve a useful purpose when it does not present difficulties.

Since the use of a tape recorder is frequently recommended throughout the voice therapy program the clinician should exercise a certain amount of care in asking children with voice disorders to listen to their own voices. Even though most children have heard their voices on a tape recorder at school or at home those recordings were usually made for fun in an uncritical situation. It is not a good idea to have a child with a severe voice problem listen to himself on a tape recorder during the first therapy session. Without proper preparation a child may be upset by the way he sounds, often refusing to listen to himself by putting his hands over his ears. The clinician should make tape recordings just for fun before doing listening training or voice analyses with a child (24, p. 114). The clinician explains how a tape recorder works and what he will hear. He is told his voice may not sound as pleasant as he would like but the use of a tape recorder will help him improve his voice.

Negative Practice

Negative practice is a very useful method in teaching good use of voice. It is the conscious use of an undesirable habit. The undesirable habit is always contrasted immediately with the desired production.

There are two steps in the use of negative practice: gross differences negative practice and fine differences negative practice. These two steps enable a child to gain conscious control of the undesirable habit and to reject the undesirable and assume the desired behavior.

Gross Differences Negative Practice

The child uses two levels of voice production, the desired and the undesired. For example in pitch problems the levels are very high pitch *versus* normal pitch or very low *versus* normal pitch. Other examples are very hypernasal *versus* normal resonance, too loud *versus* normal loudness, and very hoarse *versus* no hoarseness.

Fine Differences Negative Practice

When the child can do gross negative practice with control he is ready to do fine differences negative practice. Here three or four levels are used, for example mild, moderate, and severe hoarseness and a clear voice. When a child can gain this type of control over a faulty vocal habit contrasted to a desirable vocal habit the elimination of the undesirable becomes one of conscious choice.

The Use of Negative Practice

Negative practice is used conservatively and in limited amounts to bring undesirable vocal practices to a conscious level. It also demonstrates kinesthetic and auditory sensations of incorrect vocal production so the child can eliminate the incorrect production more easily and rapidly. Negative practice is ordinarily used only within the therapy situation. Except for special cases we do not recommend asking a child to do negative practice on voice in outside situations. This must be made very clear to a child because unsupervised negative practice may lead to overuse of this technique. When consulting with physicians about voice therapy for a child, the speech clinician should always ask about restrictions on voice therapy. Voice therapy procedures including negative practice should be explained in detail to the physician. The speech clinician must be sure it is not harmful for a child to use even limited amounts of negative practice. Negative practice may not be indicated for some children with vocal cord pathology. There may be a psychological basis for not using negative practice; it may reawaken old problems and reactions in both the child and his family (6). However, we feel carefully supervised negative practice is not harmful physically or psychologically with most types of children's voice problems.

A child is ready to begin negative practice when he can produce the desired vocal behavior. By now he has had training identifying this aspect in recordings of his own voice. For example, if we are working on a vocal abuse such as abrupt glottal attack, negative practice can begin the moment he can consciously control the abuse. He is asked to use an abrupt glottal attack on a word and then produce the word without it.

Creative dramatics and role playing including the use of hand puppets are useful in therapy (9). During the portrayal of a character we can control various aspects of a child's voice, including loudness, pitch, and quality, and pay special attention to vocal abuse. We use role playing in which a child assumes a character in his environment, especially one who may be a loud talking vocal misuser and vocal abuser. In this way a child's attention is focused on the undesirable aspects of voice production making him aware of undesirable habits. The undesirable is replaced with more desirable habits which the speech clinician teaches as the child continues role playing. Here is an example of the use of negative practice.

John, a 6½-year-old boy, had bilateral vocal nodules. His frequent use of explosive release of vocalizations was our first target for elimination. Negative practice was essential to this elimination. In his notebook we pasted pictures of things he liked and things he did not like (see Fig. 22). For example pictures of asparagus and ice cream were placed side by side. He did not like asparagus so an explosive release of vocalization was used in saying this word, while his favorite food, ice cream, was to be produced easily and smoothly. This was the first step of negative practice with only two levels used. For fine differences negative practice John used four levels for the explosive release of vocalizations—severe, moderate, mild, and normal. These types of negative practice demonstrated to John how he could control this vocal abuse and he soon eliminated it.

Habituation of New Voice Patterns

The habitual use of new voice patterns is essential for the completion of successful voice therapy. The habituation program must be planned carefully following definite procedures. Planned supervision is necessary. Per-

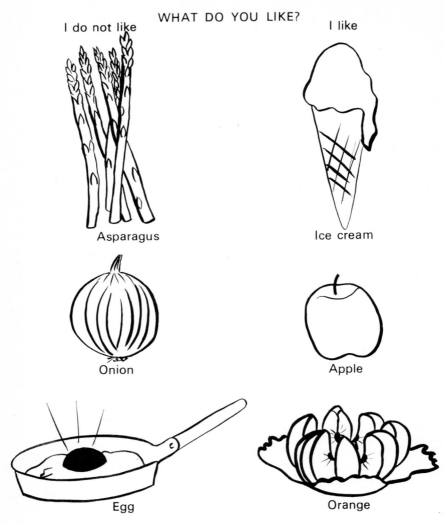

FIG. 22. Negative practice. Illustrations by Geraldine Balsam.

manent habituation must not be left to chance. The speech clinician should carefully explain the goal of each habituation assignment and have the child help plan the assignment (7). Some children find habituation relatively easy while others find it difficult. A few children have trouble using new voice patterns because the old way sounds natural to them. Any change in voice will alter this auditory monitoring sometimes with an uncomfortable feeling. A child with a soft voice may have difficulty in talking more loudly; the louder voice feels unnatural so practice is necessary for the child to get used to a new level of loudness (24, p. 113).

The child must be strongly motivated to use his new vocal patterns habitually. Several aspects of a child's voice may have been changed during the period of voice therapy. Changes may have taken place in pitch, loudness, and quality in addition to modifications of vocal abuse habits. All aspects add up to a multidimensional habituation project that requires much patience from the child, parents, and speech clinician (30). The amount of responsibility for carryover placed on a child depends upon his age. Carryover responsibility in a 4 year old is different from that of a 17 year old. The activities and instructions vary according to age, too. The younger the child the more the speech clinician depends upon other people in the environment, such as the parents and teachers, in carrying out programs to help a child habituate new voice patterns.

Structured Habituation

There are two steps in habituation: (1) limited habituation and (2) overall habituation. In limited habituation the child uses his new vocal pattern only a few minutes at a time. Assignments may include situations with the speech clinician, certain school situations, and special times at home and at play. In overall habituation the periods of carryover are extended to whole sessions with the speech clinician, class hours, mealtimes, and play periods, then to half days or evenings, and finally to the use of the new vocal pattern consistently and permanently. Each voice therapy session should provide a child with some type of carryover activity. In fact, carryover may begin with the first therapy session. As each new voice habit is taught the child immediately begins carryover. Thus at any one point he may be working on different carryover stages of several new habits.

Limited Habituation. Limited habituation is used whenever a child is introduced to a new vocal pattern. He is first asked to use this pattern only with the speech clinician and then outside the clinic in certain school situations and during special times at home and at play. Brief prearranged situations between the child and his parents or teachers should be constructed to exercise control over the new patterns (30). In some instances a new voice should be used first with strangers, then be brought into use with friends and family (28, p. 192). We feel this is especially true in cases of falsetto voices and in problems where there is quite a decided change in the voice. Later the speech clinician might ask the child to use a lower pitch when he talks to five different people at home.

Children should not be allowed to practice on their own until the speech clinician is sure they know how to do their exercises correctly (29). The speech clinician should practice each assignment with the child so it can be

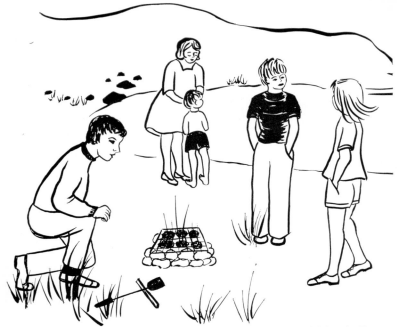

"I now use my new voice with my family and friends."

FIG. 23. Habituation. Illustration by Geraldine Balsam.

done easily and accurately; he may accompany the child on some outside situations especially those designed to practice voice control under emotional conditions or in distracting situations such as exciting games and conversations (7).

We have found the use of a notebook with the child, parents, and teachers aids in habituating new patterns. Pictures of activities with the child's family and friends can be placed in the notebook with labels "I now use my new voice with my family and friends" (Fig. 23). The notebook can be used to have a child report assignments in writing (7). When a child has learned to control certain types of vocal behavior in his daily life he should be appropriately rewarded. For young children a program of rewards can be developed with parents; older children and teenagers can develop their own system of rewards. In this way correct vocal responses can become habitual. Creative dramatics under the direction of the speech clinician aids in habituation. Creative dramatics can be used as an adjunct to speech therapy especially to bridge the gap between clinic sessions and everyday speaking. No scripts or technical aids are needed; the clinician guides the children in planning and producing the dramatization of a story or situation. Throughout the session emphasis is placed on good voice use (17).

Overall Habituation. As therapy progresses the habituation time is extended to whole sessions with the speech clinician, class hours, meal-times, play periods, then half days or evenings, and finally to overall habituation. When a child and others report the consistent use of newly learned vocal patterns carryover is complete.

To assure long term habituation of new vocal habits periodic checkups for the child should be scheduled after the concentrated voice therapy program has been completed. Appointments should be made with the speech clinician and various members of the voice team. Periodic visits to the speech clinician serve as reminders of good voice use to both the parent and child and tend to perpetuate the use of the new voice (30). Extended follow-up programs make it possible to evaluate the effectiveness of voice therapy procedures and to make sure the voice habits have become permanent.

Role of the Family in Voice Therapy

When working with children with voice problems it is necessary to enlist the cooperation of the family as supportive personnel. The parents' cooperation is essential in obtaining necessary medical, dental, and psychological examinations and treatment. The parents should be actively engaged in the voice program including evaluation, therapy, and habituation. The role of the parents during active voice therapy depends a great deal upon the type of voice problem and the type of therapy. In some situations, such as functional hypernasality, the child may need the understanding of the family concerning his problem.

In most instances when vocal behavior is being altered parents can be given specific instructions and a program worked out for their help with assignments at home. Parents may be advised of what is expected of them in different ways. Individual conferences either in person or by phone are essential at first. When written assignments are given to a child instructions to the parents can be included. Some clinics have regularly scheduled group meetings of parents to keep them informed and to discuss problems when they arise (20). In selected cases home visits are advisable (34).

The active participation of parents is especially necessary in cases of laryngeal dysfunction when vocal abuse and vocal misuse are felt to contribute not only to the original cause of the problem but also to the continuation of the problem. Parents should understand the unfavorable vocal effects of excessive screaming (16, p. 184). When a child has vocal nodules both the child and his parents should cooperate in eliminating vocal abuse (23). The successful management of vocal nodules in children requires great patience in securing family comprehension, cooperation, and motivation (1). Consideration of the psychosomatic aspects of vocal nodules necessitates not only checking the child but also his family, and in some cases therapy includes counseling for the family (34). The reduction of vocal abuse requires the concentrated effort of those involved in the child's life, including his family, teachers, and friends; the child should not be nagged but it is advisable to have an organized home program for eliminating vocal abuse (2).

A child's voice problem which is the result of imitation of others in his environment presents a real problem for the speech clinician. Counseling the child and involving the family in voice reeducation are indicated to give the child insight into the situation. If at all possible the child should be kept away from the person or other child he is imitating (14).

Special Procedures in Voice Therapy

Many children not only need learning experiences related to improvement of voice but also attention, help, and understanding of other problems which may be directly or indirectly related to the voice disorders. Behavioral training is indicated for some children with vocal nodules who are loud, boistrous, and very vocal; this includes learning to follow directions, sharing, and overcoming negative behavior (34).

Client-centered Therapy

Client-centered therapy (25) is a useful approach for helping children understand themselves (19). Thorn (27) described the use of this procedure for voice and personality problems. She stated psychological tensions, inadequate adjustment to interpersonal relationships, feelings of insecurity in social situations, long established patterns of reacting characterized by feelings of inadequacy and extreme self-consciousness may contribute to unacceptable voice patterns. This approach allows permissiveness and directs the child to the appropriate goals. The clinician sets limits on behavior. For example a child is not allowed to break toys but the clinician recognizes the child's desire to do so with understanding. Many children with voice problems are extremely active, many are overaggressive. A genuine acceptance of children by the clinician will help them understand and modify their own behavior.

Communication-centered Therapy

Communication-centered speech therapy as described by Low, Crerar, and Lassers (15) combines learning principles and therapy techniques drawn from numerous areas of human behavior. The basic tenet is the concept that communication is the nucleus for the learning of speech and the basic motivation for learning speech is to communicate not to imitate. Motivation is derived from group relationships with five general aspects which may proceed as a group begins to work together: (1) determine group and individual needs; (2) unify the group through integrating activities; (3)

plan activities which include verbal and nonverbal expression; (4) plan activities requiring new speech patterns and different behavior; (5) practice specific speech behavior in context; if necessary remove it from context for practice but always return it to the original context for further practice. If we apply communication-centered therapy to a group of children with vocal nodules, the five general aspects can be sequenced as follows: (1) define the need of the group to modify or eliminate vocal abuse identifying specific vocal abuses in each group member; (2) the group is then unified through activities such as listening training to become aware of various types of vocal abuse used by group members; (3) arrange activities which evoke communication on the vocal as well as nonvocal levels (a game in the gym or on the playground practicing controlled vocal and nonvocal communication could be arranged with the vocal abuses beginning to come under control); (4) arrange an activity requiring specific adjustive behavior on the part of the child (for example, decreased shouting would require him to adjust his behavior to a more quiet level by getting closer to people to whom he talks); (5) practice new shouting techniques in group activities as much as possible with special practice for the children who do not show adequate control of shouting in the group. Soon these children would be returned to the group situation for actual control of loudness in the original context such as a ball game.

Operant Conditioning in Voice Therapy

Operant procedures may be especially useful as a basic method in voice reeducation. These procedures, described by Skinner (26), can be applied to children with all types of voice problems. They can be used in programming instruction for a child individually or in groups.

Behavior Modification. In modifying behavior it is important to follow shaping techniques, realizing the desired terminal behavior is usually reached by a series of successive approximations. That is, when we get the initial approximation of the desired vocal response we are satisfied with this attempt and reinforce or reward the child. As therapy progresses, however, our standards become increasingly higher and a child's approximations must come closer and closer to the desired goal.

Holland (10) described two basic rules regarding approximations, "(1) Begin with a form of behavior which the learner is fully capable of emitting and (2) move rigorously and precisely in small steps from this initial performance, differentially reinforcing each step, to progressively closer approximations of the desired final behavior." She emphasized the use of shaping procedures should not be haphazard but very clearly defined and the steps worked out carefully making certain they are small enough to assure mastery.

The desired change may be either in decreasing the rate of occurrence of an undesirable response or increasing the rate of occurrence of a desirable response (5). Throat clearing may be used as an example of decreasing the rate of an undesirable response. A speech clinician may want to establish a change in the number of times a child clears his throat during a specified period. First the baseline is established; for example a child cleared his throat 25 times during a 5-min period. The allowable rate is varied so during specified 5-min periods he can clear his throat 20 times, 18 times, 15 times and so on. This definite program in reducing the number of times a child clears his throat eventually leads to extinction of this undesirable vocal habit. An example of increasing the rate of occurrence of a desirable response is substituting easy initiation of tones for abrupt glottal attacks.

Reinforcement. Brookshire (5) stated, "Operant conditioning, in its simplest sense, is the process whereby consequences . . . occur relative to a response so that the rate of the response is controlled." He presented the basic procedures in operant conditioning: (1) positive reinforcement, (2) negative reinforcement, and (3) punishment which takes two forms, presentation of an adversive stimulus and removal of a positive reinforcer. When reinforcements are used they are never delayed but are made immediately following the response (5; 10). Waiting until the end of a therapy session to place a star beside a child's name on a chart gives him little reward for any specific accomplishment other than just coming to the therapy session.

Positive reinforcement is the use of a reward for a desired response. Material consequences (soft drinks, candy, small toys, cereal, or points toward the winning of a toy) are often given for approximating or producing the desired behavior (18). Holland (10) preferred not to use these types of rewards; rather the reinforcers should be transitory so the child's attention is not distracted by eating, drinking, or playing with small toys. She preferred winning points in a game, the pleasant noise of a door chime, or other immediate, clearly distinguishable but transitory reinforcers. The child should not be so overloaded with material rewards that they become meaningless. The clinician accompanies the act of material reinforcement with the word "Good," gradually decreasing the number of times material reinforcement is used and continuing to say "Good" so that later this verbal reward is substituted for material reward. Gradually all rewards are given less frequently. This gradual withdrawal, termed fading, makes the child less dependent upon constant and frequent rewards. In this way his own modified behavior becomes the reward.

Negative reinforcement is removing an adverse or undesirable stimulus upon production of the desired response. A child is presented with a continuous undesirable stimulus which is then removed when he responds acceptably. A continuous white noise (18), a bright light, or a blindfold can be used. Negative reinforcement should be used sparingly and with care.

We seldom use these particular reinforcements because children are often uncomfortable or even frightened by them. Instead the speech clinician can use the continuous moderately intense ringing of a cowbell or buzzer either operated manually or recorded on a tape loop with the noise removed when the undesirable vocal habit is stopped or a desirable habit begun.

Punishment is the presentation of an adverse stimulus when undesirable behavior or responses occur. Examples of punishment are a sudden burst of loud noise or a bright light. This type of reinforcement can be useful in working with vocal abuse habits such as coughing and throat clearing which have no substitute behavior. Reinforcing the desired response is a better method for eliminating an undesired response with the emphasis on what to do and how to behave rather than on what not to do.

Removal of a reward is the fourth type of reinforcement. This can take two forms, either time out from positive reinforcement or response cost (18). Time out from positive reinforcement is used when the child does not respond appropriately. No response is made by the clinician, either positive or negative; reinforcement is merely stopped. Response cost can be used when a child has accumulated a certain number of material things in the way of reinforcers. When undesirable behavior occurs the accumulated material things can be taken away one at a time. When children are accumulating points in a game, incorrect responses are charged by removing points. A response cost we use is having the child pay the clinician one token each time he makes an incorrect response.

Progress and Final Reports

Progress and final reports should be prepared by the speech clinician. These require careful evaluation by the clinician. Reports become part of the child's permanent record in the speech clinician's files and copies are sent to other members of the voice team. When appropriate, copies also become part of the child's school health and academic records.

Periodic reports should be written approximately every 3 months. Sometimes it is appropriate and convenient to coincide the reports with other periodic reports such as grading periods or end of semester reports. Voice therapy reports should be brief and concise usually not more than one typewritten page. Longer reports are necessary when the child is transferred from one agency to another.

Figure 24 is the voice therapy report we use. This form was modified from one developed at The Child Guidance and Speech Correction Clinic, Jacksonville, Florida. It can be used for both periodic reports and final reports. The form contains four divisions: voice status at beginning of report period, outline of voice therapy, voice status at end of report period, and recommendations.

1. Voice Status at Beginning of Report Period. This should contain

Name of Child_____ Date of Report_____

Address _____

Voice Problem_____

Number of Voice Therapy Sessions_____ Average Length of Session_____

Date Voice Therapy Began_____ Date Voice Therapy Ended_____

    1. Voice Status at Beginning of Report Period:

    2. Outline of Voice Therapy:

    3. Voice Status at End of Report Period:

    4. Recommendations:

_____

Speech Clinician_____ Title_____

Agency_____

Address_____ Telephone_____

FIG. 24. Voice therapy report.

a basic description of the child's voice problem and ratings on the general
voice profile and special profiles at the beginning of the report period.

2. Outline of Voice Therapy. Basic and special remediation procedures are outlined. Limitations on voice use and any advice or instructions
are included.

3. Voice Status at End of Report Period. The clinician reevaluates
the child's voice by administering current voice profiles. These profiles are
reported along with the clinician's overall impression of progress. Brodnitz
(4) suggested comparing the new use of voice with previous inadequate
use by listening to tape recordings taken prior to therapy and during
therapy. Brodnitz pointed out the individual clinician may be somewhat
prejudiced in his judgment; thus we feel it is advisable to have the child's
voice evaluated by other speech clinicians also.

We like to use Brodnitz's (4) categories for determining outcome of vocal
rehabilitation: *Successful*—children who are able to produce a satisfactory
voice which reflects good physiological use, is esthetically pleasing, and
will continue to be satisfactory under varying conditions of use; *Improved*—
children who have a much improved and useable voice, but whose voice
still has some traces of the undesirable quality, pitch, or resonance; *Poor*—
children who have not obtained a better voice as a result of adequate medi-

cal and voice therapy attention; *Discontinued Treatment*—this category is for children who terminated therapy so early in the program an opinion on progress is not indicated. Brodnitz (4) in defining criteria of success in voice therapy stated both the clinician and the person himself should consider whether or not the voice therapy was a success. Many factors should be reviewed including the use a child demands of his voice. In some instances the child and his parents may be well satisfied to have an improved voice even though some undesirable aspects are still present. On the other hand, parents of a child who does a great deal of singing at school or in a choir may have higher standards regarding the results of vocal rehabilitation.

4. Recommendations. Progress reports include recommendations for continued voice therapy with considerations for change in frequency or length of sessions or for a change in the individual-group ratio, reevaluation by the voice team or any of its members, or additional examinations or tests. Final report recommendations should specify frequency of rechecks indicating the specialists to be consulted.

Some basic approaches in voice therapy have been presented. Listening training forms the basis for therapy programs. Teaching correct voice use should be systematically approached and combined with negative practice. Habituation of new voice patterns is carefully structured. The family has an important role throughout the process of vocal rehabilitation. Special procedures in voice therapy include client-centered and communication-centered therapy and operant conditioning procedures. Progress and final reports should be done periodically and sent to appropriate personnel. Next we will present voice therapy procedures for problems of laryngeal dysfunction.

REFERENCES

1. Arnold, G. E. Vocal nodules. In J. F. Daly (Moderator). Voice problems and laryngeal pathology. *New York J. Med.*, **63**, 1963, 3096–3110.
2. Baynes, R. A. Voice therapy with children: A global approach. *J. Michigan Speech Hearing Ass.*, **3**, 1967, 11–14.
3. Bindra, D., Williams, J. A., and Wise, J. S. Judgments of sameness and difference: Experiments on decision time. *Science*, **150**, 1965, 1625–1627.
4. Brodnitz, F. S. Goals, results and limitations of vocal rehabilitation. *Arch. Otolaryng. (Chicago)*, **77**, 1963, 148–156.
5. Brookshire, R. H. Speech pathology and the experimental analysis of behavior. *J. Speech Hearing Dis.*, **32**, 1967, 215–227.
6. Elliott, F. Clinical observations regarding negative practice. *J. Speech Hearing Dis.*, **25**, 1960, 196–197.
7. Engel, D. C., Brandriet, S. E., Erickson, K. M., Gronhovd, K. D., and Gunderson, G. D. Carryover. *J. Speech Hearing Dis.*, **31**, 1966, 227–233.
8. FLOWER, R. M. Voice training in the management of dysphonia. *Laryngoscope*, **69**, 1959, 940–946.
9. Hahn, E. Role-playing, creative dramatics and play therapy in speech correction. *Speech Teacher*, **4**, 1955, 233–238.
10. Holland, A. L. Some applications of behavioral principles to speech problems. *J. Speech Hearing Dis.*, **32**, 1967, 11–18.

11. Huffman, L., and McReynolds, L. Auditory sequence learning in children. *J. Speech Hearing Res.*, 11, 1968, 179–188.
12. Irwin, R. B. *Speech and hearing therapy. Clinical and educational principles and practices.* Pittsburgh: Stanwix House, 1965.
13. Karlovich, R. S. Sensory interaction: Perception of loudness during visual stimulation. *J. Acoust. Soc. Amer.*, 44, 1968, 570–575.
14. Klinger, H. Imitated English cleft palate speech in a normal Spanish speaking child. *J. Speech Hearing Dis.*, 27, 1962, 379–381.
15. Low, G., Crerar, M., and Lassers, L. Communication centered speech therapy. *J. Speech Hearing Dis.*, 24, 1959, 361–368.
16. Luchsinger, R. Physiology and pathology of respiration and phonation. In R. Luchsinger and G. E. Arnold. *Voice—speech—language. Clinical communicology: Its physiology and pathology.* Belmont: Wadsworth Publishing Company, 1965.
17. McIntyre, B. M., and McWilliams, B. J. Creative dramatics in speech correction. *J. Speech Hearing Dis.*, 24, 1959, 275–279.
18. McReynolds, L. V. Contingencies and consequences in speech therapy. *J. Speech Hearing Dis.*, 35, 1970, 12–24.
19. Martin, E. W. Client-centered therapy as a theoretical orientation for speech therapy. *Asha*, 5, 1963, 576–578.
20. Matis, E. E. Psychotherapeutic tools for parents. *J. Speech Hearing Dis.*, 26, 1961, 164–170.
21. Moore, G. P. Voice disorders associated with organic abnormalities. In L. E. Travis (Editor). *Handbook of speech pathology.* New York: Appleton-Century-Crofts, Inc., 1957.
22. Murphy, A. T. *Functional voice disorders.* Englewood Cliffs: Prentice-Hall, Inc., 1964.
23. Murphy, R. S. Hoarseness. *Nova Scotia Med. Bull.*, 46, 1967, 177–179.
24. Pronovost, W., and Kingman, L. *The teaching of speaking and listening in the elementary school.* New York: Longmans, Green and Company, 1959.
25. Rogers, C. R. *Client-centered therapy.* Boston: Houghton-Mifflin Company, 1951.
26. Skinner, B. F. *Science and human behavior.* New York: Macmillan Company, 1953.
27. Thorn, K. 'Client-centered' therapy for voice and personality cases. *J. Speech Dis.*, 12, 1947, 314–318.
28. Van Riper, C. *Speech correction. Principles and methods.* Ed. 4. Englewood Cliffs: Prentice-Hall, Inc., 1963.
29. Van Thal, J. H. Dysphonia. *Speech Path. Ther.*, 4, 1961, 11–21.
30. Wilson, D. K. Children with vocal nodules. *J. Speech Hearing Dis.*, 26, 1961, 19–26.
31. Wilson, D. K. Voice reeducation of adolescents with vocal nodules. *Arch. Otolaryng. (Chicago)*, 76, 1962, 68–73.
32. Wilson, D. K. Voice re-education of children with vocal nodules. *Laryngoscope*, 72, 1962, 45–53.
33. Wilson, D. K. Voice problems of hearing-impaired children. In *Proceedings of International Congress on Education of Deaf, Stockholm, 1970.* Saga/Svensk Lararetidning, Forlags AB, in press.
34. Withers, B. R., and Dawson, M. H. Psychological aspects. Treatment of vocal nodule cases. *Texas State J. Med.*, 56, 1960, 43–46.

5

VOICE THERAPY FOR LARYNGEAL DYSFUNCTION

Specific voice therapy procedures are indicated for children with laryngeal dysfunction with or without laryngeal pathology. The goals of voice therapy for laryngeal dysfunction are (1) eliminating or modifying vocal abuse; (2) desirable use of pitch; (3) appropriate loudness; (4) balanced muscular tonus; (5) controlled rate of speaking; (6) production of a clear voice.

These goals are adapted to each child with laryngeal dysfunction. Some children with this problem may require all six goals in a therapy program while other children may need only a few of these goals to attain improved voices. The goals constitute an overall program and are not necessarily listed in order of approach. They are the goals of the voice therapy program only and do not include the work of other team members. The basic listening training program described in Chapter 4 is essential to nearly all these goals.

Goal 1. Eliminating or Modifying Vocal Abuse

Vocal abuse must be eliminated or modified to such an extent that it is no longer considered an actual abuse (50–52). During the examination and evaluative procedures all possible vocal abuses were explored by observing the child in various school and home situations including sports and outdoor activities. The speech clinician has this record in the form of rating sheets showing how frequently each vocal abuse occurs and how vigorously it is used. The voice therapy program should be based on these ratings. It is important to reduce excessive abuse for three reasons: (1) the vocal abuse may be unpleasant and distracting to listeners; (2) modifying or eliminating vocal abuse in the absence of laryngeal pathology is a preventive measure to avoid the possibility of later development of laryngeal pathology; (3) modifying or eliminating vocal abuse often results in the reduction or elimination of a laryngeal pathology. In fact, modifying or eliminating vocal abuse assumes primacy in the program for children who have laryngeal pathology. When hoarseness is attributed to excessive and improper use of

119

the voice, improvement in voice is in direct proportion to the success in correcting vocal abuse (33).

The program for eliminating or modifying vocal abuse is based on listening training procedures and structured around the following steps. (1) The child is taught the rule about his vocal abuse. (2) The child identifies the vocal abuse in others. (3) The child identifies the vocal abuse in himself. (4) The child is taught the auditory and kinesthetic aspects of his vocal abuse. (5) The places where the abuse is used are listed. (6) The vocal abuse is eliminated *some* of the time. (7) The vocal abuse is eliminated *most* of the time. (8) The vocal abuse is eliminated or satisfactorily modified.

For each of the child's vocal abuses a chart is placed in his notebook following the program outline; for example a chart on shouting is shown in Figure 25. The chart reflects the basic approach to eliminating a vocal abuse. It can be appropriately titled for use with any type of vocal abuse. The chart is used as a progress ladder with each step rewarded as the child moves from Step 1 to Step 8. For young children small picture stickers can be placed on each rung of the ladder as he progresses from one step to another. For older children "O.K." written on the ladder is an appropriate reward.

The child is taught the rule about the specific vocal abuse (Step 1). This is done by explaining what the vocal abuse is and why it must be eliminated. The rule almost always is "Don't use the vocal abuse." The child must be informed that many of his vocal abuses are harmful to him even though other children may not suffer disastrous results from such practices. It is advisable to help the child understand his problem by giving him the

8. I DON'T SHOUT ANY MORE.   _____

7. I CAN KEEP FROM SHOUTING *MOST* OF THE
   TIME.   _____

6. I CAN KEEP FROM SHOUTING *SOME* OF THE
   TIME.   _____

5. I KNOW THE PLACES WHERE I SHOUT.   _____

4. I KNOW HOW IT SOUNDS AND FEELS
   WHEN I SHOUT.   _____

3. I CAN TELL WHEN I SHOUT.   _____

2. I CAN TELL WHEN OTHER PEOPLE SHOUT.   _____

1. I KNOW THE RULE ABOUT SHOUTING.   _____

FIG. 25. Shouting chart.

basic facts about his voice disorder and explaining the rationale for eliminating the vocal abuse (50). When appropriate the child is given an acceptable substitute activity such as whistling, blowing horns, or making other noises which do not require the use of his larynx. The notebook is useful here also. A picture representing one type of vocal abuse can be put into the notebook and labeled. On the same page another picture is placed which shows an acceptable substitute to use in this situation. For example, a picture of a boy shouting "hello" to a friend from across the street illustrates an undesirable practice and a picture of a boy waving "hello" to his friend across the street illustrates the desired way (50). Another page in his notebook can be titled "I don't have to shout to call my pets." A picture of a cat can carry the caption "I can click my tongue to call my cat" and a picture of a dog can have the caption "I can whistle to call my dog" (Fig. 26). There are no suitable substitutes for vocal abuses such as excessive talking, coughing, throat clearing, and talking in noisy places. These must be modified or eliminated. Show the child how he can clear his throat easily. Reduction of the frequency of occurrence of these abuses can be rewarded.

The child is next given listening training to learn to hear the vocal abuse in others (Step 2) and then in himself (Step 3). A page in his notebook can be titled "Do you do these things?" Pictures of his various vocal abuses can be placed on this page. For example a page may contain pictures of people shouting, screaming, cheering, and using other vocal abuses (Fig. 27). The speech clinician can sometimes bring these types of vocal abuse to the child's consciousness merely by describing them and pointing them out as they occur; other times a tape recording can be effectively used to help him identify his undesirable vocal behavior (50). Many times a throat microphone is useful in identifying undesirable auditory aspects of laryngeal habits. The microphone is attached to an amplifier and the child listens to his voice through earphones. This method can be used to identify and then modify or eliminate glottal fry, abrupt glottal attacks, excessive breathiness, pitch breaks (2), coughing, and throat clearing.

The more flagrant types of vocal abuse are relatively easy to bring to the child's attention but this may be difficult to do with certain types of abuse used involuntarily. For example the child may automatically use abrupt tone initiations as he shows enthusiasm while playing cards. Also when playing with cars, airplanes, and other toys he may automatically and unconsciously imitate the sound of the car or jet plane by producing strained vocalizations.

Next the child is taught the auditory and kinesthetic aspects of his vocal abuse (Step 4). No doubt in the process of teaching the child to identify the vocal abuse in others and in himself he began to learn the auditory aspects of his abuse. Now for example he more specifically analyzes the pierc-

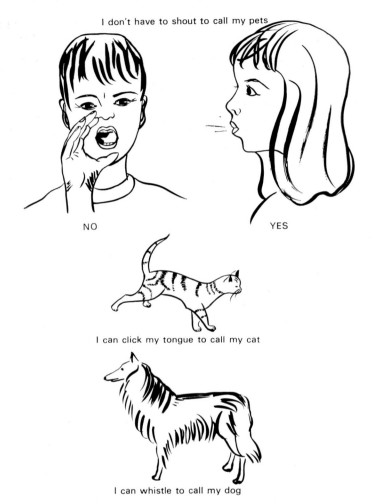

FIG. 26. Substituting nonlaryngeal sounds for vocal abuse. Illustrations by Geraldine Balsam.

ing quality of his scream and the accompanying muscular tensions in his neck, throat, and shoulders.

The speech clinician and the child discuss and identify the places or situations where the vocal abuse is used (Step 5). This is a particularly important step if his vocal abuse occurs only under certain circumstances, for example at an athletic event, on the playground, or while playing with certain toys. Recognition of the connection between abusive vocal practices and certain activites can be a big step toward eliminating the abuse.

DO YOU DO THESE THINGS?

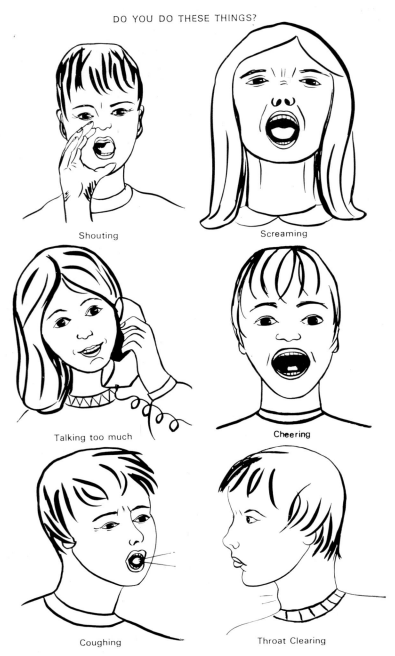

FIG. 27. Typical vocal abuses. Illustrations by Geraldine Balsam.

The three points at the top of the chart, eliminating the vocal abuse some, most, and all the time (Steps 6, 7, and 8), make up the carryover process. Activity pictures can be placed on a page in the notebook to reward the child as he begins to gain control of the vocal abuses. For example, if he or the parents report they have been on a picnic and certain vocal abuses were not used, a picture of a family on a picnic titled "I can have fun with my family and not shout or scream" is appropriate (Fig. 23).

The general plan outlined above can be adapted to handle the different vocal abuses, shouting, screaming, cheering, excessive talking, strained vocalizations, reverse phonation, explosive release of vocalizations, abrupt glottal attack, throat clearing, coughing, and talking in noise. Additional techniques for the more common vocal abuses follow.

Cheering

The child or youth should be taught to attain loudness without strain. Cheering by teenagers at sports events is especially difficult to curb. Uris (44) presented a program to teach the teenager to cheer, taking the major muscular strain off the vocal cords and transferring it to the abdominal muscles which can stand strain. Uris suggested the following exercises to be used with groups of teenagers. (1) Breathe in rhythm and on inhalation take a deep breath. The low abdominal wall, not the chest, should expand on inhalation and then contract on exhalation. The group breathes in unison and upon signal says /hɑ/ several times. (2) Cheer with syllables beginning with /h/: /haɪ/, /ho/, /hi/; /haɪ/, /ho/, /hi/. (3) The /b/ is dropped and the group chants vowels without the /h/, attempting to retain the same release feeling as with the /h/. (4) Each teenager places his hands on his abdomen, takes in an easy deep breath, and then cheers /rɑ/, /rɑ/, /rɑ/. With each /rɑ/ the abdominal wall contracts and then relaxes. "Without any forcing from the throat, the cheer grows more and more vigorous and with enough volume to please the most rabid fan."

Strained Vocalizations

The elimination of the child's use of strained vocalizations to imitate the sounds of cars or planes may require special techniques. Turn on the tape recorder and play a racing car game with the child with car noises represented by strained vocalizations by both child and speech clinician. Play the recording, teach the identifying features of the abuse, and then have the child tally his own and the clinician's strained vocalizations. Go through the same procedure again but this time substitute the strained vocalizations with easy vocalizations, whistling, or vibrating the lips. A page in the notebook can have a picture of a child with his mouth open (with NO written under it) and a child pursing his lips as if they were vibrating (with a YES written under this picture). The page can have pic-

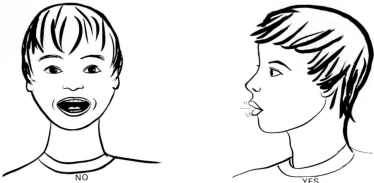

NO   YES

I don't have to make sounds with my voice when I play with my toys.
I can blow air through my lips and still make a lot of noise.

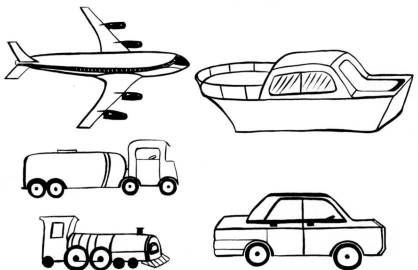

FIG. 28. Eliminating vocal abuse. Illustrations by Geraldine Balsam.

tures of cars, planes, boats, trains, and trucks with the couplet "I don't have to make sounds with my voice when I play with my toys, I can blow air through my lips and still make a lot of noise" (Fig. 28). The eight steps on the chart can be followed to eliminate this abusive practice and achieve carryover of substitute activities.

Explosive Release of Vocalizations and Abrupt Glottal Attack

Special attention must be paid to eliminating explosive vocalizations and abrupt glottal attacks. Reducing the force of abrupt glottal attacks is of great importance in obtaining ease of vocal cord adductions (35). Teaching easy breathing for speech is particularly recommended when abnormal vocal attacks are found in a person who has vocal nodules (8, p. 213; 38; 47, p. 192). Brodnitz (15) suggested breathing exercises when there is definite need to reduce the pressure of the breath against the vocal cords to teach adequate release of air during phonation.

Listening training is useful in teaching a child correct vocal attack to replace explosive or abrupt glottal attacks. The speech clinician demonstrates abrupt and easy attacks for the child discussing the characteristics of each. The child identifies these attacks as they appear in the clinician's demonstration. The child then is taught to use relaxed phonation (30, p. 691). This can be done by using the three steps of teaching correct vocal practice. The first two steps, awareness and gross discrimination, can be handled according to instructions in Chapter 4. The third step, fine discrimination of differences in his own voice, may require special handling for this type of problem. In learning a normal vocal attack the child usually overdoes it and produces a breathy attack. This can be incorporated into the fine discrimination practice. The three productions for fine discrimination, then, are abrupt glottal attack (or explosive release), the desired normal attack, and breathy attack. In this way the child learns to identify and eliminate both forms of undesirable attack and adopts the normal attack.

Laryngeal tension during abrupt glottal attacks should receive special attention. Have the child place the tip of his finger on the triangle of the thyroid cartilage as he uses an abrupt attack. The tension will be reflected in the elevation of the larynx. The child can then be shown that vocalizing in a relaxed easy manner results in little or no elevation of the larynx (49, p. 218). Brodnitz (14, p. 93) recommended the chewing method for reduction of abrupt glottal attack. This method will be described in connection with achieving balanced muscular tonus.

Negative-positive practice helps teach the child to modify his abrupt attacks to softer, easier initiations. A useful technique for this is the "clothespin-feather" game, using negative-positive practice techniques. A child emits an abrupt tone as he vigorously throws a clothespin into a large metal container. The clatter of the clothespin as it hits the bottom of the container is associated with his abrupt attacks. Then the child is asked to modify his abrupt attacks to easy initiations. Prolonging continuant consonants (17) or beginning with an /h/ or breathy attack (30, p. 693; 34, p. 11) helps prevent an abrupt attack. This time he drops a feather into the container as he uses an easy attack. The slow movement of the feather and its easy landing in the container are likened to the new easy tone initiation. Listening to tape recordings of this activity is useful in establishing the identification of easy tone initiation.

We have used exercises similar to those listed by Rubin and Lehrhoff

(39) to teach children correct attack on sounds. These can be copied and placed in his notebook.

1. Make believe you are yawning and breathe out easily as you say the vowels /ɑ/, /o/, and /u/. Then say them easily without a yawn. Breathe in deeply and sigh as you let the air out and say a vowel sound as you gradually lower the pitch.

2. Remember to talk quietly with a good voice. Also talk clearly. Read a story or a poem in a quiet voice.

3. Whisper the vowels /ɑ/, /æ/, /i/, and /o/. As you do each one change the whisper to a good tone.

4. Say vowel sounds with an /h/ in front of each one. Be sure to say them easily with good tones. Get a list of words beginning with /h/ from your dictionary. Practice saying them easily. Then omit the /h/ in all words that still make a real word, such as hat/at or hold/old. Practice the new words easily with good tones.

The child's notebook can be used as a visual aid in working on tone initiation. A page titled "Easy Voice" may contain three pictures of waves hitting a shore representing "easy," "hard," and "very hard" tone initiation. The size of the waves represents the three types of tone initiation. The child names each picture using the three types of initiation. Phrases and sentences for each picture can also be used. Prolonging initial sounds aids in developing a smoother less interrupted flow of tone.

All vocal abuses should be worked on until they are eliminated or so modified that they are no longer considered abusive vocal practices. With many children eliminating vocal abuse ends traumatizing practices which caused a laryngeal pathology or dysfunction. A better voice is the dividend. Following is an example of a child in whom reduction of excessive talking and eliminating other vocal abuses were the major goals of voice therapy (adapted from Wilson (52)).

Terry's kindergarten teacher referred him to the speech clinic because he talked too fast and too loudly and had a hoarse voice. The medical report from the family physician described him as an essentially normal child in development and general physical condition. The child had always talked in a loud voice, and the parents had been unable to get him to talk with less intensity. They reported that he talked constantly at home and during play, although the mother denied excessive yelling or screaming. He occasionally became hoarse when he was fatigued, but never aphonic. Voice tests revealed a child with a hoarse, breathy voice with many pitch breaks and abrupt, hard initiation of tones. He talked loudly and excessively, using long sentences, and he was readily intelligible. Audiometric testing revealed normal hearing.

The child was referred to a laryngologist for consultation because of the hoarseness. Examination of the vocal cords showed small vocal nodules at the junction of the anterior and middle thirds of each cord. It was felt that the nodules in all probability were due to improper use of the voice and also that the cords became more swollen as the day went on when he used his voice a great deal. The laryngologist noted that the child was very talkative and loud. He felt the nodules were too small for removal, and that voice training was indicated, especially if the child could be quieted down to a moderate degree. Psychological examinations revealed a child with adequate emotional maturity with normal intelligence.

During a period of 3 months the boy was seen for a series of 16 sessions with the speech clinician. When voice therapy was initiated his voice was hoarse in a moderate degree rated 5 with much vocal abuse noted, such as excessive loud talking and forced high-pitched sounds made in play activities. The conversational voice was not abnormally high in pitch; therefore, voice therapy was designed only to reduce the amount of talking and to eliminate other vocal abuse. A laryngeal examination following voice therapy indicated the nodules were significantly reduced in size, and it was the impression that hoarseness had been practically eliminated. He was no longer abusing his vocal cords or talking as much. The laryngologist observed that the vocal cords did not seem to hit each other as abruptly and hard as they had prior to voice therapy. Subsequent voice evaluations over a period of a year following voice therapy revealed the voice to be clear and free from hoarseness.

Goal 2. Desirable Use of Pitch

The results of the pitch examination should be studied carefully before considering changes in pitch use. Recommendations for changing an habitual pitch level should not be made indiscriminately (13) but are made only after careful evaluation. Children and adolescents exhibiting unsatisfactory use of pitch generally fall into one or more of the following five classifications: (1) pitch problems related to mutation, involving a high pitch level in the adolescent male or an unusually low pitch level in the adolescent female (appropriate changes in the habitual pitch level are in order for these problems); (2) excessive pitch breaks usually associated with voice change (these should be eliminated); (3) frequent use of traumatizing high or low pitch levels under certain circumstances, such as in games and outdoor activities even though the habitual pitch level and pitch range are adequate under normal speaking conditions, also some children may use abnormally high pitch while speaking loudly under noisy conditions or talking under emotional strain (if these abnormal pitch levels are used enough to be considered damaging children should be taught to avoid even the intermittent use of unusually high or low pitch levels); (4) the habitual continuous use of too high or too low pitch levels considered to be traumatizing and contributing to the laryngeal dysfunctioning (changes in habitual level are indicated); (5) stereotyped and limited voice range (instruction for improved expression is indicated for these problems).

Pitch is not an isolated factor of the vocal characteristics of a person (14, p. 96). Teaching overall good use of voice in its various parameters of loudness, inflection, and quality often results in a suitable habitual pitch level. For example, we know a decrease in loudness lowers pitch and an increase in loudness results in a higher pitch. Also, teaching a child to talk in an easier fashion rather than in a staccato, hard manner with abrupt attacks modifies his use of pitch to a more acceptable level without paying direct attention to the pitch of his voice.

Perkins (36, pp. 870–871) stated any tone requiring strain to produce is undesirable whether it is high or low, but tension is less likely to be present when the voice is produced near the bottom of the range than when it is produced near the top of the range. He objected to the practice of mechanically analyzing the voice for the habitual and optimum pitch levels and deciding to change pitch if there is an appreciable difference between the levels. He felt these measurements are sometimes invalid because of tension in the vocal cords resulting from increased subglottal air pressure. He favored a more subjective approach in which the person is encouraged to use as low a pitch as is comfortable to get a voice production that is effortless and free from tension.

Laguaite and Waldrop (28) stated as a general rule pitch should not be worked on directly but advocated therapy techniques for easy relaxed phonation. They stated the fundamental pitch of a person's voice should not be changed unless it is significantly different from the norm established for that particular age. They compared mean fundamental frequencies and acoustical analyses of subjects before and after therapy. They found the fundamental frequency did not change significantly but the acoustical analyses indicated more vocal energy in the higher frequencies and greater regularity in the harmonics. Therefore, they concluded that changes in voice as a result of therapy are due to factors other than changes in fundamental frequency.

The habitual pitch of a child's voice should not be changed unless it is necessary. We feel a change in habitual pitch level may be indicated when the habitual level is considered to be traumatizing and is contributing to the particular laryngeal dysfunction present. This is especially true in children with vocal nodules, thickened vocal cords, chronic nonspecific laryngitis, and hyperkeratosis. In many cases adequate use of pitch may be obtained through manipulation of other factors such as changing loudness or working on balanced muscular tonus while speaking.

A change in pitch level is often necessary for children and adolescents with vocal nodules (52) because of the necessity to change the area of vocal cord contact (8, p. 213). West and Ansberry (49, p. 217) stated that in patients with vocal nodules relief must be given to the rubbing edges of the vocal cords by moving the point of greatest friction. They felt the pitch ordinarily should be lowered since vocal nodules usually result from the use of too high pitch. They based therapy on the following principles. (1) The point of maximum friction between the vocal cords moves from back to front as the pitch rises. (2) There is at least one level, and in adult males possibly two levels, of pitch best for the person. When pitch is placed at this point there is more efficient phonation. This is the point at which loud tones can be made without damage to the vocal cords. Above and below this ideal or optimum pitch a person is required to force his voice using a great amount of air pressure. (3) There must be a reduction of this air pressure during phonation to lessen the friction between the vocal cords. The location of the nodules may give an indication of the pitch level being used incorrectly. If the nodules are anterior one can assume the pitch has been too high and high pitches should, therefore, be avoided (49, p. 217). Thus a child with vocal nodules located at the junction of the anterior and middle thirds of the vocal cords usually needs to have the habitual pitch level lowered to the norm for his age.

Children with other laryngeal conditions may need normalizing of the pitch. No doubt all children with laryngeal dysfunction should be taught to avoid intermittent use of very high or very low pitch levels even though the habitual pitch level is normal. In general we feel a speech clinician should be very discriminating in his therapeutic use of pitch change unless the child deviates significantly from the norm for his age and sex.

Changing Pitch

Changes in pitch can be achieved by administering a thorough program of listening training and then teaching correct pitch level and pitch variability. The listening training sharpens pitch discrimination ability and prepares the child for specific control of pitch. The basic outline for listening training can be used here. Awareness of differences in pitch in the clinician's voice and gross discrimination on two levels can be covered quickly. The speech clinician can then concentrate on fine discrimination of three levels— high, middle, and low. These three pitch levels are based upon the child's pitch range and habitual pitch level. If the child's pitch is too high, the clinician selects a high level near the top of the range which often coincides with the too high habitual level. The middle pitch is carefully selected as the level to be established as the new habitual level. The third level is a low level only slightly above his lowest pitch. The child is told the significance of each level: the high level is the old way to be avoided, the middle is the desired new way, and the low pitch is too low to use most of the time (50).

Pictures for pitch practice can be placed in the notebook. For example the speech clinician can use a picture of three children standing at different

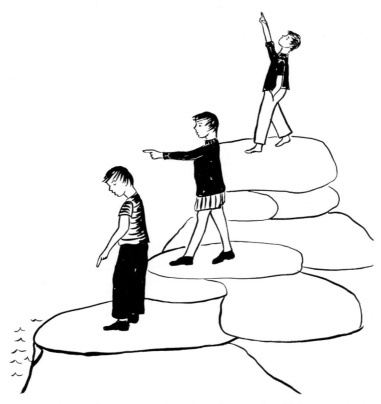

FIG. 29. Pitch practice representing three levels—too high, correct, too low. Illustration by Geraldine Balsam.

heights on rocks. These can be labeled "I can talk low," "I can talk in the middle," and "I can talk high" (Fig. 29). The speech clinician demonstrates the three levels with words, phrases, and sentences for discrimination training with the child pointing to the appropriate figure.

Another technique for pitch training is called the space game (50). The speech clinician places three pictures of airplanes in the child's notebook, one at the top of the page, one in the middle, and one at the bottom. These are captioned "high airplane," "middle airplane," and "low airplane," and the three pitch levels are repeatedly demonstrated by the clinician and associated with each picture. When the child has begun to categorize pitch into the high, middle, and low levels the speech clinician makes up stories about the three pictures and keeps changing pitch levels. Each time the level changes the child points to the appropriate picture. Pictures of birds, rockets, or balloons can also be used.

Practice by the child himself follows listening training when he has developed good pitch discrimination. The roles of the child and the speech clinician are reversed with the child becoming the performer and the clinician the listener and judge. The child knows from his listening training the significance and meaning of the three levels of pitch and can therefore strive to produce each pitch level. The pictures used to develop discrimination can be used for the child to practice the pitch levels. Other useful devices for identifying and establishing proper use of pitch level involve simple skits in which the child is encouraged to use the three pitch levels in impersonating characters. Puppets can be used as the basis for these skits.

The pitch chart (Fig. 30) is to be used by the child in a manner similar to other charts. The chart is placed in his notebook and each step rewarded appropriately as he progresses up the ladder.

Robby, a 6½-year-old boy, is an example of pitch misuse causing vocal nodules. Lowering the habitual pitch level resulted in a normal laryngeal mechanism. He was referred to the speech clinician by a laryngologist with the complaint of hoarseness and the diagnosis of "screamer's nodes" about 2 mm in size bilaterally at the junction of the anterior and middle thirds of the vocal cords. About 1 year prior to the referral the child had a series of colds and two attacks of bronchitis, and it was then that the parents began

9. I CAN TALK WITH THE CORRECT PITCH
   ALL THE TIME.   _____

8. I CAN TALK WITH THE CORRECT PITCH
   MOST OF THE TIME.   _____

7. I CAN TALK WITH THE CORRECT PITCH
   SOME OF THE TIME.   _____

6. I KNOW THE PLACES WHERE I USE THE
   CORRECT PITCH.   _____

5. I KNOW THE PLACES WHERE I USE THE
   WRONG PITCH.   _____

4. I CAN HEAR THE CORRECT PITCH IN MY
   VOICE.   _____

3. I CAN HEAR WHEN THE PITCH OF MY
   VOICE IS WRONG.   _____

2. I CAN TELL WHEN OTHER PEOPLE USE
   HIGH AND LOW VOICES.   _____

1. I KNOW THE RULE ABOUT THE PITCH OF
   MY VOICE.   _____

Fig. 30. Pitch chart.

to notice the hoarseness. This hoarseness continued after recovery from the colds, however, and became increasingly worse. He was a very active boy with more hoarseness at the end of a day of hard playing and yelling. He habitually talked excessively in a loud voice with a high pitch level. He continually abused his vocal cords by using strained high-pitched sounds in play activities. The pediatrician felt that the boy was developing normally and was generally in good physical condition. The child was doing well in the first grade and was a leader among his peers.

Voice tests indicated the child's voice was hoarse in a severe degree (#6) with the conversational voice generally dysphonic and at times aphonic especially at the ends of breath groups. There was no hoarseness on sustained vowels when the voice was pitched 2 to 3 semitones below the habitual level. A psychological evaluation revealed a child with adequate social adjustment and average intelligence.

The laryngologist and the speech clinician conferred on the case, and it was decided to give the child voice training for a period of 3 months. Accordingly, the child was seen by the speech clinician for 17 sessions. The objectives of voice therapy included: (1) lowering the habitual pitch of the voice, (2) reducing the amount of loud talking and yelling done in a high pitch, and (3) eliminating the hoarse voice quality. After 3 months of training by the speech clinician the second laryngeal examination revealed a significant reduction of the nodules beyond that expected under normal procedures without voice therapy. Voice training was continued for an additional 9 sessions over a period of 4 months. At the conclusion of these sessions vocal abuse was modified, the habitual pitch was lower and the voice practically free from hoarseness. A third laryngeal examination at this time indicated the nodules were no larger than a pinhead. The child was placed on a bimonthly voice check with the speech clinician. A fourth laryngeal examination 14 months after the initial one revealed that the nodules were no longer present. The voice was clear, the lower habitual pitch was being used, and subsequent rechecks by the speech clinician over a period of 3 years indicated the child was free from any symptoms of hoarseness (adapted from Wilson (52)).

Disturbed Mutation of the Voice

Treatment should be instituted for disturbed mutation when boys are in their teens or at the latest in their early twenties because if the falsetto voice persists there may be some atrophy of the vocal muscles because of disuse (48). The speech clinician will find cases of delayed or partial mutation and persistent falsetto voice in high school boys. Very infrequently boys have precocious vocal mutation, that is, sexual maturity with a low-pitched voice beginning before age 8 (29, p. 197). Perverse mutation is also infrequent; that is when the female voice changes into an abnormally low-pitched voice upon puberty. Even though the speech clinician sees very few with the last two problems, it is necessary to recognize them and be prepared to handle them.

The speech clinician can begin a program to change the habitual pitch level in a teenager if the laryngologist's examination reveals normal laryngeal structures and general normal functioning. However, voice therapy is also indicated when laryngeal irritation is felt to be due to disturbed mutation. Psychotherapy should be synchronized with voice therapy when indicated.

Voice therapy for delayed or partial mutation or a persistent falsetto voice follows the general outline of voice therapy procedures. First, it is necessary to give the youth a structured program of listening training. This follows the three major steps of listening training, awareness of differences, gross discrimination, and fine discrimination of differences in others. When discrimination between the high pitch and the desired lower pitch has been established, the young man can be taught to produce the lower pitch level voluntarily (16). We first make sure he is aware of his own incorrect pitch levels through tape recordings of his voice compared to recordings of the desired pitch levels.

Then we teach him to produce a correct pitch level. This usually can be done quite quickly in only a few sessions, sometimes in the first session. The adolescent can often be taught a new lower pitch by having him imitate the lower pitch of a male speech clinician; it is sometimes useful to amplify the clinician's voice by funneling it directly into the boy's ear (16). Another method of obtaining normal pitch and quality of voice in cases of falsetto voice is to have the boy first produce a vocal fry in isolation and then in softly spoken speech (1). Luchsinger (29, p. 196) described a useful method. The boy is instructed to hum a sustained tone. The speech clinician presses the thyroid cartilage inward and downward. The pressing inward relieves excessive contraction of the cricothyroid muscle. A low-pitched voice emerges almost automatically. Then the boy is taught to lower the pitch voluntarily without touching the larynx.

When the boy can produce the desired pitch we work to establish this pitch level. We introduce negative practice by having the boy produce his old high pitch and contrast it to the new low pitch. When he can do this we ask him to experiment with three levels of pitch, too high, correct, and too low. Bryngelson (16) suggested the following steps in establishing the use of the desired pitch level in adolescents. Practice reading aloud under supervision with the speech clinician restimulating the new lower pitch when necessary. Then proceed to nucleus situations where the new lower pitch is used for only a few sentences beginning with very short sentences. Then the boy is asked to use his new low pitch in social situations. Then he may be asked to do limited negative practice outside the clinic to gain voluntary control over the undesirable high pitch level. Soon he can be asked to tabulate the number of times the old high pitch level is used in outside situations.

Frequently a boy is reluctant to use the new pitch level in outside situations. A marked change in voice can be traumatic to an individual because it may be a surprise both to the individual himself and to his associates (47, p. 229). This type of patient, as well as his mother, first rejects the new low voice and persuasion may be necessary for permanent carryover (29, pp. 196–197). If there is too much resistance psychotherapy should accompany voice therapy (21, p. 197; 48).

The therapy principles we wish to emphasize regarding treatment of falsetto voice are best illustrated by the following case history.

Kevin was referred to us by his high school public speaking teacher during his junior year in high school. He was 17 years of age, a tall, slender, masculine-appearing young man, one of the top basketball players in high school. The basketball coach was preparing him for his senior year when he was expected to bring state honors to the high school basketball team. In a preliminary interview we found his habitual pitch level was approximately 280 Hz when talking with normal loudness. During louder talking his habitual pitch went up to over 300 Hz. He reported he had not experienced any type of voice change during puberty and he was now becoming concerned about his voice. He stated he was occasionally teased about his high-pitched voice but since he was well known in the school it was generally accepted. He stated his most embarrassing times occurred when he answered the telephone and the caller thought he was a girl. He readily admitted one of the reasons he concentrated on athletics was in an effort to express his masculinity. Kevin reported he dated frequently, attending most of the social functions at the school with his steady girl friend. We requested a laryngological consultation. The laryngologist assured us all laryngeal structures were of normal size and function. The school physician assured us of Kevin's normal physical maturation and secondary sex characteristics. Psychological testing by the school psychologist included intelligence tests and various projective techniques. The test results were summarized by the school psychologist as follows: above average intelligence, a normal heterosexual adolescent without any deviant personality patterns. The psychologist noted strivings to prove himself to be masculine, probably mainly as compensation for his high-pitched voice. Following these tests the laryngologist, school physician, psychologist, and speech clinician met to discuss the results of the tests and to formulate a treatment program for Kevin. The group felt if the habitual pitch of this adolescent could be lowered through voice therapy most of his problems would be solved. Voice therapy was recommended three times a week for half hour sessions. During the first voice therapy session through singing and experimenting with various pitch levels good vocal tones were isolated at approximately 135 Hz. During the next three sessions the new low pitch was used on nonsense syllables, words, phrases, and sentences. During the fifth session Kevin conversed with the speech clinician in his new low pitch. Kevin was reluctant to try his new voice outside the clinic so we planned a gradual habituation program. We began carryover by having Kevin use his new low voice while making phone calls from the clinic room to stores and other places where he was not known. Kevin was particularly reluctant to use his new voice at home. With his permission we talked with his parents to arrange situations so he could use his new low voice without surprise from them or his brother and sister. Kevin described his therapy experiences to them using his new voice. We devised a situation in Kevin's speech class where he could give a talk about his voice therapy program; this was appropriate because the general topic under discussion was personal improvement of speaking habits. As he began his speech he was to use his old habitual high pitch and as he explained the various techniques we had used he planned to demonstrate how he first lowered his pitch on an isolated vowel. He planned to increase his use of the new pitch during his speech so that by the time he finished talking he was using his new low pitch continuously. Kevin came to the clinic after class to report on his speech and used his new low pitch to the clinic secretary before he came into our office. He had completely sold the class on his new voice. Fortunately many members of the basketball team were in the class so at basketball practice that afternoon he used his new low pitch. We saw Kevin every other week for 3 months and then for an occasional check-up during the rest of his high school career. His new low voice became permanent.

Pitch Breaks

Both boys and girls are apt to go through a period during mutation characterized by many voice breaks. After this problem has been evaluated by the laryngologist and the speech clinician a program of voice therapy is planned. An adolescent should not strain his voice during the period of voice change. He should follow good voice hygiene principles by avoiding vocal abuse and vocal misuse. Van Riper (46, p. 166) stated control of pitch breaks can be taught fairly easily. He suggested the use of negative practice through deliberately practicing the pitch breaks. This helps make the youngster feel less self-conscious about pitch breaks. The youth should be cautioned against developing tension in the laryngeal area in an attempt to avoid pitch breaks. If laryngeal tension is present the speech clinician may need to follow some of the suggestions for achieving balanced muscular tonus (Goal 4).

Goal 3. Appropriate Loudness

Most children with laryngeal dysfunction habitually talk too loudly. In these cases it is important to eliminate loud talking. This is especially true of children with vocal nodules (50; 52). Even in the absence of laryngeal pathology we are interested in reducing excessive loudness present on an habitual basis as a preventive measure to avoid possible pathological changes in the larynx. Loudness usually can be reduced quite readily in a direct manner with special attention to habituating the softer voice (36, p. 869). In fact, in some cases learning to talk more distinctly decreases the necessity to talk loudly (47, p. 192).

Modifying Loudness

The pattern for loudness listening training is similar to that used for pitch and in some cases pitch and loudness training can be combined (50). It is necessary for the speech clinician to develop awareness of excessive loudness or softness in speech intensity and then proceed to gross discrimination. For fine discrimination of loudness four loudness levels are selected: (1) a very high speech intensity approximating a shout, (2) high speech intensity termed very loud, (3) a level or range of loudness calculated to be most desirable or just right for the child to use under most circumstances, and (4) low speech intensity considered to be too soft. Pictures are placed in the notebook representing these four levels of loudness. These can be pictures of children using these loudness levels (Fig. 31). Another technique for loudness listening training is called the animal game (50). The clinician selects four pictures of animals ranging from very large to small in size to represent the four loudness levels. As with pitch training the child is asked to point to the correct picture as the clinician uses various intensity levels.

After listening training has resulted in good discrimination of loudness the child is ready to demonstrate his own ability at controlling speech intensity. The loudness chart (Fig. 32) is used for loudness modification and control. As with similar charts picture stickers or simply a written "O.K." may be used as rewards. An amplifier with earphones such as an auditory training unit can be used in teaching voice monitoring especially adequate control of loudness (12; 47, p. 259). If we want a child to talk softer we turn the volume control up and he automatically decreases his loudness level. The reverse can be done in order to increase voice loudness. Feeding a masking noise into the child's ears through earphones also increases the loudness of his voice. The masking noise from an audiometer or a recorded white noise on a tape loop can be used. Careful listening training has to accompany these techniques for carryover from the auditory trainer or amplifier into conversational use. All these activities should be tape recorded for the child to listen to so he can learn to monitor his own voice. During the recording the child can watch the recorder's intensity meter or light and listen to his own loudness levels when he is engaged in these activities with the clinician (51). The pictures in Figure 31 can be used by the child for practice.

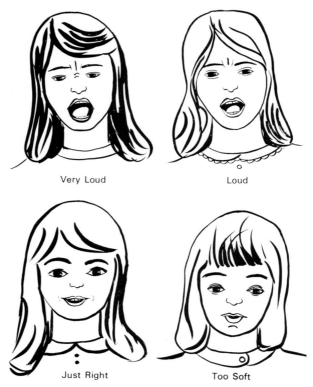

Very Loud   Loud

Just Right   Too Soft

Fig. 31. Loudness practice. Illustrations by Geraldine Balsam.

The intensity of the speech clinician's voice can be expected to influence the intensity of the child's responses (3; 9; 10; 24). The greater the intensity of a speaker's voice the greater will be the intensity of the listener's vocal response. Therefore, when we are working upon modifying the intensity of a child's voice we can expect an increase in the loudness of his responses if we talk louder to him; in contrast, softer talking by the speech clinician will result in a decrease in the loudness of the child's voice.

Black (11) found soft speech was accompanied by a slower rate while reading phrases. Some children may use an excessively slow rate at a low level of loudness. Increasing rate of talking may help bring the loudness to a more normal level.

Loudness training, even though an uncomplicated procedure, requires careful application of the listening training program, followed by teaching the correct level of loudness through auditory and kinesthetic cues reinforced by visual displays. Control of loudness is very important in maintaining good vocal hygiene and is an essential element in voice improvement.

10. I CAN TALK WITH THE CORRECT LOUD-
NESS *ALL* THE TIME.   _____

9. I CAN TALK WITH THE CORRECT LOUD-
NESS *MOST* OF THE TIME.   _____

8. I CAN TALK WITH THE CORRECT LOUD-
NESS *SOME* OF THE TIME.   _____

7. I KNOW THE PLACES WHERE THE LOUD-
NESS OF MY VOICE IS CORRECT.   _____

6. I KNOW THE PLACES I TALK TOO LOUDLY.   _____

5. I CAN TELL WHEN THE LOUDNESS OF MY
VOICE IS CORRECT.   _____

4. I CAN TELL WHEN MY VOICE IS TOO LOUD. _____

3. I CAN TELL WHEN OTHER PEOPLE HEAR
MY LOUD TALKING.   _____

2. I CAN TELL WHEN OTHER PEOPLE HAVE
LOUD VOICES.   _____

1. I KNOW THE RULE ABOUT LOUD TALKING.   _____

Fig. 32. Loudness chart.

Singing

Improper singing can be a vocal misuse if pitch or loudness is misused during singing. Both boys and girls should avoid singing during voice change (48). The singing of all children should be carefully supervised, but caution is particularly important if laryngeal pathology is present. Improper use of the voice in singing should be avoided, especially when a hoarse voice is purposely used and a breathy style combined with excessive exertion, strain, and loudness (31). The loud raucous rock style of singing, particularly when young men extensively use falsetto, can result in traumatic laryngitis and bilateral vocal cord nodules (6).

As a general rule if vocal pathology is present the child should be excused from singing until his voice has improved and the pathological condition has cleared up or significantly improved. Singing should be eliminated in cases with vocal nodules until the nodules are resolved and then it can be resumed but with different techniques (4; 26; 36). If the youngster with vocal nodules is allowed to continue vocally unrestrained in singing class he will develop irreversible vocal changes (26). Disturbances of the voice may not be apparent during speaking but become apparent during singing, for example subtle variations in vocal quality, the appearance of voice breaks, and the complaint of discomfort in the throat and neck during or following singing (38). We suggest the speech clinician and the singing teacher coordinate their efforts with children who have good speaking voices but have alterations in vocal quality during singing. The singing teacher may improve faulty singing techniques while the speech clinician concentrates on the speaking voice.

We are not specifically concerned with the professional singer, but many singers do have nodular thickenings or even polypoid thickenings of the cords that apparently do not keep them from making a good living and probably account for the distinctive character of their singing voice (4).

Goal 4. Balanced Muscular Tonus

Production of an adequate voice is based upon a balance of muscular tonus not only in the laryngeal area but also in the neck, shoulders, and, in fact, the whole body. Hyperfunction (overtense muscle tonus) and hypofunction (overly lax muscle tonus) are to be avoided. The concept of relaxation should be replaced with well adjusted tonus (14, p. 90). Proper tensions and timing in the musculature of the larynx and pharynx (18, p. 218) are basic to good laryngeal tones. It is necessary to modify or eliminate faulty vocal habits especially those producing excessive tensions (32, p. 110). In cases of vocal nodules it is important to develop general freedom from tension especially of chest, throat, and facial muscles. Freedom from tension in the extrinsic laryngeal and pharyngeal musculatures is a goal in therapy for harsh voices (47, pp. 223–224).

Hypofunction is the basis of nonorganic voice problems involving flaccid adjustments of the vocal mechanism which result in breathiness. This may require a different approach than voice disorders due to hyperfunction (36, p. 858). Thus our discussion under this goal is divided into two sections: (1) therapy for hyperfunction and (2) therapy for hypofunction. Normalizing the muscular tonus prevents all types of vocal abuse and often results in adequate use of pitch (15) and loudness without paying specific attention to these latter two voice parameters. Hyperfunction usually causes a higher pitch and hypofunction may cause an abnormally low pitch.

Hyperfunction

The correction of hyperfunction is one of the most important goals in vocal rehabilitation (14, p. 90). Perkins (36, pp. 859–862) stated the person should be taught the kinesthetic sensations of an efficient voice and the feeling of getting the throat open and relaxed for efficient voice production: "The efficient voice . . . feels as cool and open and big as a sigh." In contrast he stated the inefficient voice is like an automobile being driven with the brakes on, with both the brakes and the motor straining during forward movement of the automobile; instead the person should feel as if his voice is coasting.

Exercises to Reduce Hyperfunction. Many techniques can be used for children with hypertense vocalization. The purpose of these techniques is to achieve reduction of generalized tension in the entire body and specifically in the laryngeal area, neck, and shoulders. For problems of hoarse voice relaxation to modify the upward displacement of the larynx is recommended (47, p. 239). For problems of ventricular phonation of a nonorganic nature the speech clinician should obtain lowering of the thyroid cartilage during phonation and relaxation of the suprahyoid muscles in order to get sustained tones without laryngeal tension (47, p. 220). Training in good posture is helpful in reducing hypertension of the extrinsic muscles of the larynx and pharynx of persons with vocal nodules (47, p. 193). Breathing exercises can sometimes be helpful in relieving tensions of muscles in throat and neck areas (25). For young children rag doll games can be useful to teach the child the sensation of reduced tension during speaking. With older children and adolescents more formal exercises may be indicated. Five exercises listed by Rubin and Lehrhoff (39) have proved useful in obtaining properly adjusted tonus of muscles.

1. Have the child sigh very gently to feel the openness of the throat. Have him yawn deeply with the mouth opened as wide as possible.

2. Ask the child to tense the large muscles of the body and then suddenly relax. Point out the different muscular sensations of contraction and relaxation.

3. Do progressive muscle relaxation. Have the child relax the fingers first, then the hands, arms, body, and legs. Soft soothing background music may help the child relax.

4. Have the child roll his head forward and then around his shoulders in a slow circle as he says vowel sounds smoothly and easily.

5. Teach the child to tighten the muscles at the back of the neck. Have him move the head backward in a tense fashion. Then have him move the head from side to side, and then forward. Repeat the same exercise with relaxed easy movements, pointing out the difference in tension between the two.

Exercises Using Speech Sounds. Perkins (36, p. 865) suggested having the person sigh very gently, transform it into a whisper, then into a soft breathy tone. He emphasized that pitch should be kept at a comfortable level. After the person can phonate with a half-whispered tone the fullness should be gradually increased until he has clear nonbreathy phonation with adequate pitch and loudness. Vowels, diphthongs, or nonsense syllables can be used. The vowel /ɑ/ can be used to develop awareness of full tones and /ɔɪ/, /aɪ/, /e/, and /i/ to get a sense of openness, better projection, and vitality (36, pp. 866–867). Drills in sustaining voiced continuant consonants help to relieve hypertension centered around the laryngeal area (17).

The Chewing Method. The chewing method is sometimes effective for persons with hyperfunctional voice problems. This method has been used for some time in Europe and was described by Froeschels (20) and Froeschels and Jellinek (22, pp. 179–180). This method can also be used in mutational difficulties and to correct voice problems of the deaf and hard of hearing (21). Brodnitz (14, pp. 90–93) regarded Froeschels' method as the best way to correct hyperfunction and to reduce abrupt glottal attack. He felt (14, p. 96) an important by-product of the chewing method is the normalizing influence it has on pitch of the voice.

We have used the chewing method with children with hyperfunctional voice problems and have found it to be successful in reducing hyperfunction and in obtaining good clear tones. Following is a description of the chewing method applied to a child.

1. The child is told he can talk and chew at the same time using the same muscles for both functions.

2. The child is requested to chew without anything in his mouth with the lips closed but with energetic movements of the tongue and lips. During this activity the child is asked to be especially conscious of the movements of his tongue.

3. The child is asked to chew "like a savage" (20) with an open mouth and with very vigorous movements of the lips and tongue. Special attention should be given to obtaining good tongue movement.

4. The child is asked to vocalize while he is chewing. The speech clinician should make sure this is not just a monotonous noise but includes many different sounds.

5. The child is asked to chew with vocalization about 20 times a day for a few seconds each time. It is helpful if he keeps in mind he is pretending he has food in his mouth.

6. After several days of this chewing activity he should begin to read aloud after each session of vocalized chewing.

All chewing should be done pretending food is in the mouth and actual food or gum chewing is not advocated (21). With this method it may be possible to obtain some very good sounds free of the voice deviation and at a pitch suitable for the child without paying direct attention to quality or pitch. The child can be made aware of the clear tones and contrast them to his old way of talking. Recording these two qualities can be done for listening practice. We have found this can be fun for the child but all efforts should be made to keep the activity of chewing free from silliness.

Hypofunction

Hypofunctional voice problems are characterized by excessive breath escape, weak laryngeal tones, low speech intensity, and low pitch levels. Inadequate glottal closure is also found in children with vocal palsy and laryngeal hypofunction due to trauma to the larynx as well as in problems of functional breathy voices. In some laryngeal problems such as chronic nonspecific laryngitis the voice is too breathy with a weak glottal attack and a voice of low intensity. With breathy voices it is necessary to reduce the amount of wasted air to achieve a better voice pattern (47, p. 235). Exercises to overcome flaccid laryngeal muscle activity have been suggested in the treatment of hysterical aphonia (5). Velopharyngeal insufficiency is often caused by hypofunctioning velar and pharyngeal muscles.

Exercises to Increase Muscular Tonus. To overcome hypofunction, Van Riper and Irwin (47, p. 237) suggested asking the person to initiate vocalization suddenly and strongly perhaps initially employing abrupt tone initiation to do this. To obtain clear phonation they suggested having a person hold his breath against strong abdominal contraction and then suddenly explode the tone. We have found in working with a child with a breathy voice this technique is a good one. We ask the child to stand against a wall while the clinician presses on the child's abdomen asking him to maintain a steady pressure against the clinician's hand as the child says vowels, words, and sentences. This technique usually if not always results in good clear tones. The clear tones are tape recorded and contrasted to the breathy tones for listening training.

In a breathy voice with excess waste of air during phonation Curtis (18, p. 226) suggested asking the child to phonate in a louder tone thus increasing muscular tonicity resulting in elimination of breathiness. When the child hears the difference between the breathy and clear tones, the loudness of his voice can be reduced to an appropriate level making sure the breathiness does not return (18, p. 226). Another method of reducing breathiness is to note its occurrence on the plosive sounds /p/, /t/, and /k/. Canfield (17) stated these sounds are apt to be more breathy than other sounds and this breathiness is carried over into the following sounds. He stated it is necessary for the speaker to be made aware of his breathiness of these sounds; more precise articulation of these particular plosives will often reduce a generalized breathiness of all sounds.

Pushing Method. Froeschels' pushing exercises are useful in increasing muscle tonus to eliminate hypofunction (23). Brodnitz (14, pp. 94–95) discussed correction of hypofunction through the use of Froeschels' pushing exercises. He stated correction of hypofunction presents a particularly difficult problem for the speech clinician. He recommended pushing exercises to get more muscular activity in cases of incomplete glottal closure during phonation. It is also used to obtain improved velopharyngeal closure especially in cases of velar paralysis (23). The objective of the pushing method is to get more activation and firmer closure of the vocal cords as well as improved velopharyngeal closure. Pushing exercises consist of simultaneous movements of the arms and phonation (23). To do this a child stands and raises his fists to his chest and then pushes his arms down in one quick sweep with the hands opening just as the palms land on the front of the thighs. When this can be done without undue tension the child is requested to say vowels using /ɑ/ first and then proceeding to other vowels. Vocalization is initiated at the beginning of the downward movement and ends as the palms hit the thighs. When a good voice has been produced on the vowels, syllables and monosyllabic words are used. Five to ten pushes should be done every half hour on the 1st day and once an hour daily for a week (23). The number is then reduced according to vocal progress. As laryngeal tone and loudness improve ask the child to say a sound, syllable, or word during the pushing movement and to follow this immediately with a repetition of the vocalization without pushing but matching the volume and tone of the pushed vocalization. When good phonation develops the actual movements can be stopped with the person only thinking of pushing while he is speaking or reading aloud. These exercises energize the whole body including the voice and speech producing mechanisms. In the beginning stages vocalizations may need to be initiated abruptly in order to get a clear tone free from breathiness. Very soon, however, these abrupt initiations should be modified to easy initiations to avoid possible trauma to the larynx.

Goal 5. Controlled Rate of Speaking

Many children with laryngeal dysfunction have problems in the rate of speaking. They may speak too rapidly or too slowly. A rate problem also exists if there is lack of variation in rate or if staccato speech interferes with good voice production (49, p. 278). Faulty use of the vocal mechanism related to laryngeal hyperfunction may be accompanied by an excessively rapid rate of speaking. It is difficult to detect and change traumatic and damaging vocal habits in a child who talks too fast; this is especially true if he uses abrupt glottal attacks along with a rapid, staccato style (53). Thus, attaining an adequate rate of speaking in cases of laryngeal dysfunction is necessary (35).

Therapy for Rate

When a child's rate has been judged to be too rapid he must first be made aware of his rapid rate by listening to tape recordings of his speech comparing his recordings with pretaped samples of slow, average, and fast rates. Then his rate of speaking can be reduced to a desirable pace through oral reading and speaking exercises which stress suitable rate, correct use of pauses, and good vocal inflections (53). Rate can be reduced by using correct duration of sounds in words (43, p. 225) and using adequate phrasing and smoothness (37, p. 111). Rate may also be reduced by increasing pause time between words, phrases, and sentences (43, p. 225).

Altered breathing patterns may cause rate problems. Curtis (18, pp.

217–218) noted that breathing exercises in themselves need not be used for most cases, but if there is insufficient breath for phrases of normal length corrective drills and exercises can be used to lengthen phonation time in talking without the necessity of stopping to inhale frequently. This training makes certain a child has adequate breath reserve for good voice and gives a child the secure feeling of having sufficient air for talking (25).

A study was made of the speaking rate of a group of children aged 5 to 7 (40). A clown head made of papier mâché with a red light for a nose was used as the reinforcing apparatus. The children were told to talk to the clown to make him happy and his nose would light up. This caused the rate of the children's speech to increase. If we wish to reduce a child's rapid rate of speaking we can reverse this process. That is, the clown would be unhappy with a rapid rate and would turn off the red light. A slower rate would be reinforced by turning on the light. A simple device like this could be used with the speech clinician operating a hidden switch.

The speaking rate chart (Fig. 33) is used in a fashion similar to voice charts. The child is taught the rule about proper rate. He learns to identify slow and fast rate in others. He knows when his rate is too slow or too fast

9. I CAN TALK WITH THE CORRECT RATE *ALL* THE TIME.   _____

8. I CAN TALK WITH THE CORRECT RATE *MOST* OF THE TIME.   _____

7. I CAN TALK WITH THE CORRECT RATE *SOME* OF THE TIME.   _____

6. I KNOW THE PLACES WHERE THE RATE OF MY SPEECH IS CORRECT.   _____

5. I KNOW THE PLACES WHERE MY SPEECH IS TOO SLOW OR TOO FAST.   _____

4. I KNOW WHEN THE RATE OF MY SPEECH IS CORRECT.   _____

3. I CAN TELL WHEN MY SPEECH IS TOO SLOW OR TOO FAST.   _____

2. I CAN TELL WHEN OTHER PEOPLE'S SPEECH IS TOO SLOW OR TOO FAST.   _____

1. I KNOW THE RULE ABOUT HOW FAST I SHOULD TALK.   _____

Fɪɢ. 33. Speaking rate chart.

and he knows the correct rate for himself. He knows the places where his rate is incorrect and where it is correct. Carryover from partial to complete habituation follows. Action pictures are placed in the child's notebook. He is asked to tell stories about them as he practices slow, fast, and correct rate of talking. For example he can tell a story about the dog (Fig. 34) varying his rate according to the picture being described.

Goal 6. Production of a Clear Voice

Obtaining a clear and resonant voice is a major goal in voice therapy for laryngeal dysfunction (35). Teaching adequate vocal patterns usually begins with the first session and is done concurrently with the elimination of inadequate vocal patterns. That is, as an inadequate pattern is being eliminated it is replaced by an adequate pattern. This rule applies to all vocal rehabilitation procedures except those vocal abuses which must be eliminated when there are no suitable substitutes.

Eliminating vocal abuses, teaching the proper use of pitch and loudness, establishing balanced muscular tonus, and controlling rate of speaking often result in a clear laryngeal tone with good voice resonance. With some children, however, additional procedures may be necessary to develop a voice free from the undesirable laryngeal characteristics. A good voice chart (Fig. 35) can be placed in the child's notebook to keep track of his progress in improving quality. This chart is used in the same manner as the charts previously presented. The rules about a clear voice are explained. He is told he must first learn to recognize a hoarse voice in others and in himself. Next he will learn how to produce a good voice and use this voice instead of the old one. A concentrated program of listening training is the first step. This precedes direct attempts to improve laryngeal tone.

Listening Training for Improved Laryngeal Tone

The initial step of listening training, awareness of differences, is approached first. The child indicates when the clinician produces sounds with excessive breathiness, harshness, or hoarseness. A principal technique for developing gross discrimination of differences is called the bad-good game (50). The top half of a page of the child's notebook is designated the "bad" part and the bottom half the "good" part. Related pictures are pasted on the "bad" and "good" halves. A picture of an outlaw on the bad half is described by the clinician in a voice that is an imitation of the child's quality and a picture of a marshal on the good half is described in a voice free from hoarseness. The child is asked to point to the picture indicated by the quality being used by the clinician. Similar stories can be centered about the "bad and good" technique. When the child can identify both the presence of clear and defective laryngeal tones produced by the clini-

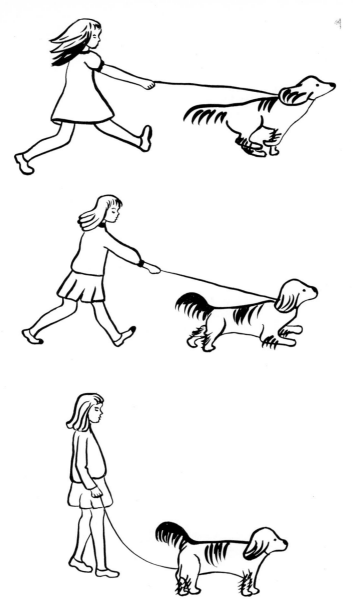

Fig. 34. Rate practice representing three levels—too fast, correct, too slow. Illustration by Geraldine Balsam.

9. I CAN TALK WITH A CLEAR VOICE *ALL* THE TIME

_____

8. I CAN TALK WITH A CLEAR VOICE *MOST* OF THE TIME.

_____

7. I CAN TALK WITH A CLEAR VOICE *SOME* OF THE TIME.

_____

6. I KNOW HOW IT FEELS WHEN I TALK WITH A CLEAR VOICE.

_____

5. I KNOW HOW IT FEELS WHEN I TALK WITH A HOARSE VOICE.

_____

4. I CAN HEAR WHEN MY VOICE IS CLEAR.

_____

3. I CAN HEAR HOARSENESS IN MY VOICE.

_____

2. I CAN TELL WHEN OTHER PEOPLE HAVE HOARSE VOICES.

_____

1. I KNOW THE RULES ABOUT CLEAR VOICE.

_____

FIG. 35. Good voice chart.

cian he is rewarded by having a sticker placed on Step 2 of the good voice chart, "I can tell when other people have hoarse voices."

The third step in listening training, fine discrimination of differences, is next approached. Pictures of the three palm trees (Fig. 36) can be used for this step. The pictures are labeled "clear," "rough," and "very rough." The child designates the quality being used by the clinician by pointing to the correct picture.

An important adjunct in the listening training of children is to have them listen and judge their own performance from recordings. Samples obtained during the examination can be used. The child listens to these recordings which contain samples of sounds or words, some of which have clear laryngeal tones and some defective laryngeal tones. When the child correctly identifies the instances of hoarse and clear quality he is rewarded for Step 3 on the chart "I can hear hoarseness in my voice" and Step 4, "I can hear when my voice is clear." When listening training is well under way the child is ready to be taught to produce a better voice.

Locating a Satisfactory Tone

Special techniques are necessary to discover good tones in some children. Voice scanning techniques described by Van Riper and Irwin (47, p. 286) are useful as a basis for teaching improvement of voice. They suggested

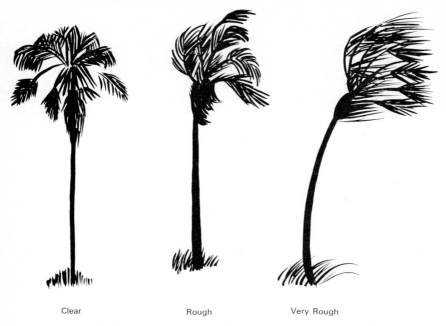

Clear   Rough   Very Rough

FIG. 36. Voice quality practice. Illustration by Geraldine Balsam.

finding the child's new voice by having him go through the whole repertoire
of possible phonations to locate the desired tones. Good vocalization can
usually be found by varying loudness or pitch levels on vowels or words.
After the child has found an acceptable voice he then is taught the auditory
and kinesthetic images of this voice. It is usually necessary to use progressive approximations to obtain a better voice with the person being encouraged as he more closely approximates the desired voice (46, p. 190).

A method we use for finding a good tone is as follows. (1) Have the child
assume a good standing posture where he is at ease, perhaps against a wall
where he has some support. (2) Have the child breath through his nose, the
clinician places a finger above the larynx. (3) Have the child sustain a good
/m/. The tone should come through the nose with good resonance and with
the throat open and relaxed. The larynx should not move upward; the neck
muscles in particular should be relaxed. (4) The child initiates a good /m/
in this manner at various pitch levels. (5) Have the child phonate a good
/m/ as he did in Step 3 with throat open, no upward movement of the
larynx, neck muscles relaxed, and then have the child open his mouth to
produce the sound /ɑ/. The sound should be soft at first and then gradually increased in loudness with repeated production. Practice all the vowels
in this manner. (6) The acceptable vowels are combined with other initial

consonants for syllable drill and then practiced in nonsense syllables where consonants both precede and follow the vowel. Exercises using words, phrases, and sentences follow. During these exercises emphasis should be placed on clarity of sounds, correct pitch placement, adequate loudness, and good resonance.

Production of improved quality by the child can be based on imitation if it is done under expert guidance and a good voice is selected as the ideal (36, p. 874). For example, a binaural amplifier can be used with the child's voice fed into one of his ears and the clinician's voice into the other ear or both voices into the same ear.* Van Riper (45) stated the clinician can begin blending his voice to match that of the child, speaking in unison, repeating words or sentences several times. The clinician then gradually modifies the stimulation, introducing variations toward the desired pitch or voice quality. When this is done correctly the child follows the slight gradations until a more normal voice results. As a result of using these techniques some children are able to produce good tones free from laryngeal deviations. With other children we are able to obtain improved tones which need additional attention.

Procedure for Improving Tones

Teaching adequate stress on words improves voice quality and eliminates forced tones (41). Have the child sing to obtain a continuous flow of phonation being sure he uses an appropriate pitch level and firm articulation (41). Attention also should be paid to lengthening and strengthening voiced continuant consonants such as /z/, /v/, and /l/; sometimes prolonging or giving due phonation time to these types of consonant sounds eliminates breathiness and harshness (41). These sounds should be sustained for two rhythmic beats or counts as a person talks to obtain better and stronger phonation (17). When this added time is given to the voiced continuant consonant sounds the articulators develop more tonicity and sounds become clearer as well as more accurate (17). Emphasis should be placed on obtaining an easy voice production that is free from strain and excessive loudness. This can be aided by having the child take an easy breath and use an easy voice, making sure that an adequate breath supply is maintained while talking (7).

In some instances negative practice helps a child produce an improved voice. For example, in the case of hoarseness the child listens as the speech clinician demonstrates both desirable quality and hoarseness on vowels, words, and phrases. The hoarseness does not necessarily have to be an exact imitation of the child's hoarseness but should approximate it. The child is then asked to repeat the same vocalizations alternating his usual

---

* Binaural Speech Trainer, HC Electronics, Inc., Tiburon, California 94920.

hoarse quality with as clear a voice as possible. This is recorded and played back on a tape recorder and the child is requested to evaluate the success of his attempts at producing a clear voice.

We should pay attention to the excessive dropping of the mandible in speaking. In a radiographic study Shelton and Bosma (42) found when their subjects had a wide opening of the mouth the tongue was quite consistently humped and the pharyngeal airway was reduced in some subjects. In studying the pharyngeal airway with various head positions they found a wide opening of the mouth produced the greatest airway reduction. In contrast they found while a lax opening of the mouth resulted in some reduction of the pharyngeal diameter this was less extensive than during the wide mouth opening. With a lax opening tongue humping was not observed. They found the dorsal portion of the tongue is apparently the ". . . key mobile pharyngeal element in airway regulation. Its strategic role is indicated by the multiplicity of its function. It regulates the airway in the mesiopharynx and in the laryngeal vestibule, and it rises to approximate the soft palate."

Canfield (17) stated that excessive or wide excursions of the jaw add to reduced tongue tip activity which results in poor voice quality. To increase tongue tip activity for improved voice quality he recommended the person be told to hold his upper and lower teeth lightly together during practice periods, thus forcing the tongue to move more. He stated attention to precision of articulation during this type of practice will result in better oral, nasal, and pharyngeal resonance. Thus if we say to a person, "Open your mouth more" or "Move your jaw more" we may be promoting inadequate tongue tip activity and a reduction of the pharyngeal airway. This may result in poor articulation and poor voice quality. We should be very cautious in giving these commands unless the child actually has an inadequate mouth opening and little jaw movement.

When a child can produce good tones he progresses up the voice chart to Step 4, "I can hear when my voice is clear." When he has learned the kinesthetic sensations of hoarse and clear voice production he continues up the ladder through Steps 5 and 6.

Carryover is sometimes difficult in establishing permanent use of good voice habits. A child may have difficulty making use of new voice patterns because he is accustomed to his old way of talking and the new voice sounds and feels strange to him. However, practice in using new vocal patterns gradually adjusts him to his new voice. Steps 7, 8, and 9 on the voice chart are used as the child progresses from partial to complete use of his new voice.

Ventricular Phonation

Ventricular phonation presents a special problem requiring special techniques. Thus a separate section on this problem is appropriate. In a very few instances the true cords may be absent or deformed. For these cases ventricular phonation must be continued and this substitute voice should be trained to function as well as possible (14, p. 77). In cases where the true cords are present with the possibility of normal functioning, the goal of voice therapy is to eliminate the ventricular phonation tranferring this phonatory effort to the true cords. The person should be taught to speak at an optimum pitch and learn to control the laryngeal muscles so true vocal cord vibration can be encouraged and the vibration of the false vocal cords decreased and eliminated (19). Van Riper and Irwin (47, p. 221) felt that if the speech clinician regards the problem of ventricular phonation as a respiratory abnormality more success is assured. Sometimes voiced inhalation prior to regular phonation brings the true vocal cords into use. They (47, p. 221) also have found that initiating tones using a glottal fry helps mobilize the true vocal cords. Children with ventricular dysphonia present on a psychogenic basis respond well to voice therapy especially when it is combined with encouragement and discussions regarding the basis of the disturbance. Progress in this type of problem is slow and it may be necessary to have a period of prolonged supervision in order to prevent recurrences; in severe cases psychiatric consultation should be sought (14, p. 77).

We have found all these techniques useful in working with cases of ven tricular phonation, but one approach we have found most useful is a program of listening training combined with direct teaching of an improved voice. This is illustrated by the following case example (54).

A physician noticed during a routine physical examination that this 14-year-old girl had an extremely hoarse voice. This hoarseness had been present consistently since infancy. She was very self-conscious and often refused to talk because she was teased about her low hoarse voice quality. The physician referred her to a laryngologist who diagnosed the disorder as dysphonia plicae ventricularis neonatorum—a congenital anomaly in which phonation is accomplished by the ventricular bands instead of the vocal cords alone (27, p. 31). A voice evaluation by the speech clinician revealed the girl could use the true vocal cords alone in phonating several vowel sounds of good quality. These vowels and several hoarse vowels were recorded so the girl could contrast the two qualities. Beginning with this listening training she was taught to use the true vocal cords more and more and to eliminate ventricular phonation. She received voice therapy for 4 months. A laryngeal examination 8 months after the original one revealed adequate action of the vocal cords and elimination of the phonatory movement of the ventricular bands. This child was fortunate in that the true vocal cords were present. When the true cords are absent on a congenital basis a low-pitched and hoarse voice using the false vocal cords may be the maximal that can be obtained.

Rules for a Good Voice

This chapter can be summarized by presenting rules for a good voice for children with laryngeal dysfunction. A set of rules should be made up for each child according to his particular vocal abuse and vocal misuse. These rules can be written in a child's notebook in terms he can understand and can be illustrated with pictures appropriate for his age. Select from the following list the rules that apply to a particular child.

1. Talk quietly. Whistle or use noisemakers instead of shouting, screaming, and cheering. Whistle or click your tongue to call pets. Wave your hand to say "hello" to people far away.

2. Avoid using reverse phonations, strained vocalizations, explosive release of vocalizations, or abrupt glottal attack.

3. Talk when you wish, but not too much. Do not give oral reports in class, act in plays, do public speaking, or sing until your physician and speech clinician approve.

4. Clear your throat easily.

5. Cough only when you really need to and do it easily.

6. Avoid talking in noisy places—like around machinery, riding in an auto at high speeds, or when listening to loud music.

7. Talk at the correct pitch level—not too high or too low.

8. Talk at the correct loudness level—not too loud or too soft.

9. Talk easily without straining the muscles in the throat, neck, and shoulders.

10. Talk at the correct rate—not too fast or too slow.

REFERENCES

1. Anonymous. Helpful hints. *W. Mich. Univ. J. Speech Ther.*, 1, 1964, 6–7.
2. Anonymous. Clinical helps. *W. Mich. Univ. J. Speech Ther.*, 3, 1966, 11.
3. Atkinson, C. J. Vocal responses during controlled aural stimulation. *J. Speech Hearing Dis.*, 17, 1952, 419–426.
4. Baker, D. C., Jr. Laryngeal problems in singers. *Laryngoscope*, 72, 1962, 902–908.
5. Bangs, J. L., and Freidinger, A. Diagnosis and treatment of a case of hysterical aphonia in a thirteen-year-old girl. *J. Speech Hearing Dis.*, 14, 1949, 312–317.
6. Batza, E. M. Vocal abuse in rock-and-roll singers. Report of five representative cases. *Cleveland Clin. Quart.*, 38, 1971, 35–38.
7. Baynes, R. A. Voice therapy with children: A global approach. *J. Michigan Speech Hearing Ass.*, 3, 1967, 11–14.
8. Berry, M. F., and Eisenson, J. *Speech disorders. Principles and practices of therapy.* New York: Appleton-Century-Crofts, Inc., 1956.
9. Black, J. W. The intensity of oral responses to stimulus words. *J. Speech Hearing Dis.*, 14, 1949, 16–22.
10. Black, J. W. A compensating effect in vocal responses to stimuli of low intensity. *J. Exp. Psychol.*, 40, 1950, 396–397.
11. Black, J. W. Relationships among fundamental frequency, vocal sound pressure, and rate of speaking. *Lang. Speech*, 4, 1961, 196–199.
12. Brodnitz, F. S. Contact ulcer of the larynx. *Arch. Otolaryng. (Chicago)*, 74, 1961, 70–80.
13. Brodnitz, F. S. The holistic study of the voice. *Quart. J. Speech*, 48, 1962, 280–284.
14. Brodnitz, F. S. *Vocal rehabilitation.* Ed. 3. Rochester, Minn.: American Academy of Ophthalmology and Otolaryngology, 1965.
15. Brodnitz, F. S. Rehabilitation of the human voice. *Bull. N. Y. Acad. Med.*, 42, 1966, 231–240.

16. Bryngelson, B. The functional falsetto voice. *Speech Teacher*, **3**, 1954, 127–128.
17. Canfield, W. H. A phonetic approach to voice and speech improvement. *Speech Teacher*, **8**, 1964, 42–46.
18. Curtis, J. F. Disorders of voice. In W. Johnson and D. Moeller (Editors), *Speech handicapped school children*. Ed. 3. New York: Harper and Row, 1967.
19. Fred, H. L. Hoarseness due to phonation by the false vocal cords: Dysphonia plicae ventricularis. *Arch. Intern. Med. (Chicago)*, **110**, 1962, 472–475.
20. Froeschels, E. Hygiene of the voice. *Arch. Otolaryng. (Chicago)*, **38**, 1943, 122–130.
21. Froeschels, E. Chewing method as therapy. *Arch. Otolaryng. (Chicago)*, **56**, 1952, 427–434.
22. Froeschels, E., and Jellinek, A. *Practice of voice and speech therapy. New contributions to voice and speech pathology*. Boston: Expression Company, 1941.
23. Froeschels, E., Kastein, S., and Weiss, D. A. A method of therapy for paralytic conditions of the mechanisms of phonation, respiration and glutination. *J. Speech Hearing Dis.*, **20**, 1955, 365–370.
24. Hanf, C., and Corso, J. Intensity of the voice and the theory of activation. *Amer. J. Psychol.*, **79**, 1966, 226–233.
25. Hauth, L. Voice improvement: The speech teacher's responsibility. *Speech Teacher*, **10**, 1961, 48–52.
26. Holinger, P., Johnston, K. C., and McMahon, R. J. Hoarseness in infants and children. *Eye, Ear, Nose, Throat Monthly*, **31**, 1952, 247–251.
27. Jackson, C. Anomalies of the larynx. In G. M. Coates and H. P. Schenck (Editors), *Otolaryngology*. New York: Harper and Row, 1967.
28. Laguaite, J., and Waldrop, W. F. Acoustic analysis of fundamental frequency of voices before and after therapy. *Folia Phoniat. (Basel)*, **16**, 1964, 183–192.
29. Luchsinger, R. Physiology and pathology of respiration and phonation. In R. Luchsinger and G. E. Arnold. *Voice—speech—language. Clinical communicology: Its physiology and pathology*. Belmont: Wadsworth Publishing Company, 1965.
30. Moore, G. P. Voice disorders associated with organic abnormalities. In L. E. Travis (Editor), *Handbook of speech pathology*. New York: Appleton-Century-Crofts, Inc., 1957.
31. Moses, P. J. Pathology and therapy of the singing voice. *Arch. Otolaryng. (Chicago)*, **69**, 1959, 577–582.
32. Murphy, A. T. *Functional voice disorders*. Englewood Cliffs: Prentice-Hall, Inc., 1964.
33. Orton, H. B. The significance of hoarseness. *New Orleans Med. Surg. J.*, **103**, 1951, 511–515.
34. Peacher, G. Voice therapy for ulcers and nodules of the larynx. In *Proceedings of the first institute on voice pathology, and the first international meeting of laryngectomized persons*. Cleveland Hearing and Speech Center, 1952.
35. Peacher, G. M. Voice therapy. In J. F. Daly (Moderator), Voice problems and laryngeal pathology. Symposium and Panel Discussion. *New York J. Med.*, **63**, 1963, 3104–3107.
36. Perkins, W. H. The challenge of functional disorders of voice. In L. E. Travis (Editor), *Handbook of speech pathology*. New York: Appleton-Century-Crofts, Inc., 1957.
37. Pronovost, W., and Kingman, L. *The teaching of speaking and listening in the elementary school*. New York: Longmans, Green and Company, 1959.
38. Rubin, H. J. Role of the laryngologist in management of dysfunctions of the singing voice. *Trans. Pacif. Coast Otoophthal. Soc.*, **45**, 1964, 57–77.
39. Rubin, H. J., and Lehrhoff, I. Pathogenesis and treatment of vocal nodules. *J. Speech Hearing Dis.*, **27**, 1962, 150–161.
40. Salzinger, S., Salzinger, K., Portnoy, S., Eckman, J., Bacon, P. M., Deutsch, M., and Zubin, J. Operant conditioning of continuous speech in young children. *Child Develop.*, **33**, 1962, 683–695.
41. Scholl, H. M. A holistic approach to the teaching of voice improvement. *Speech Teacher*, **10**, 1961, 200–205.

42. Shelton, R. L., Jr., and Bosma, J. F. Maintenance of the pharyngeal airway. *J. Appl. Physiol.*, **17**, 1962, 209–214.
43. Strother, C. R. Voice improvement. In J. M. O'Neill (Editor), *Foundations of speech*. New York: Prentice-Hall, Inc., 1941.
44. Uris, D. Teen talk. *Todays Speech*, **10**, 1962, 15–16.
45. Van Riper, C. Binaural speech therapy. *J. Speech Hearing Dis.*, **24**, 1959, 62–63.
46. Van Riper, C. *Speech correction. Principles and methods.* Ed. 4. Englewood Cliffs: Prentice-Hall, Inc., 1963.
47. Van Riper, C., and Irwin, J. V. *Voice and articulation.* Englewood Cliffs: Prentice-Hall, Inc., 1958.
48. Weiss, D. A. The pubertal change of the human voice. *Folia Phoniat. (Basel)*, **2**, 1950, 127–158.
49. West, R. W., and Ansberry, M. *The rehabilitation of speech.* Ed. 4. New York: Harper and Row, 1968.
50. Wilson, D. K. Children with vocal nodules. *J. Speech Hearing Dis.*, **26**, 1961, 19–26.
51. Wilson, D. K. Voice re-education of adolescents with vocal nodules. *Arch. Otolaryng. (Chicago)*, **76**, 1962, 68–73.
52. Wilson, D. K. Voice re-education of children with vocal nodules. *Laryngoscope*, **72**, 1962, 45–53.
53. Wilson, D. K. Voice re-education in benign laryngeal pathology. *Eye, Ear, Nose, Throat Monthly*, **45**, 1966, 76–80.
54. Wilson, D. K. Voice therapy for children with laryngeal dysfunction. *Southern Med. J.*, **61**, 1968, 956–958.

6

VOICE THERAPY FOR RESONANCE PROBLEMS

This chapter contains a discussion of hypernasality and hyponasality present on an organic or functional basis. Therapy is designed for hypernasality due to velopharyngeal insufficiency caused by cleft palate or a variety of structural, muscular, or nerve disabilities in the velopharyngeal area. This voice problem may also be present on a functional basis with a normal velopharyngeal mechanism improperly used. Therapy for hyponasality will also be presented.

Nasal sounds have been found to constitute approximately 11 % of the phonemes in speech, /n/ 6.43 %, /m/ 3.16 %, and /ŋ/ 1.27 % (23). We can expect nasal consonants to be present in normal connected speech at an average rate of more than 1 per sec, assuming phonemes are produced at the rate of 10 per sec (9). If a child also nasalizes some of the oral sounds the impression of hypernasality is indeed marked. Therefore it is important to correct undue nasality on non-nasal sounds. A single therapeutic approach to those with hypernasal voices due to developmental disturbances is inadequate; in some cases developmental disturbances of the tongue require attention to lingual maneuverability, while others without the tongue involvement need little if any of this type of attention (8). The clinician must know the specific cause of the hypernasal voice to plan appropriate voice therapy procedures.

The goals of voice therapy for problems of velopharyngeal insufficiency are as follows. The particular goals used for a specific child depend upon his needs as revealed by the results of the diagnostic tests and examinations. (1) Improving articulation ability and increasing speech intelligibility; (2) developing adequate oral breath pressure and oral air flow; (3) improving voice quality; (4) eliminating facial grimaces and nares constriction; (5) modifying or eliminating vocal abuse and establishing balanced muscular tonus; (6) establishing adequate use of loudness, pitch, and speaking rate.

156

Goal 1. Improving Articulation Ability and Increasing Speech Intelligibility

The correction of articulation errors reduces nasal emission of sounds and decreases hypernasality (4, p. 673). Improving speech intelligibility also aids in decreasing hypernasality. McWilliams (12) in studying adults with cleft palate speech found a correlation of .720 between intelligibility scores and nasality ratings. A correlation of .821 was found between consonant articulation errors and nasality ratings. This correlation indicates when consonant errors are reduced there will also be a reduction in nasality.

All defective sounds should be approached through a well organized program of articulation remediation. The speech clinician should review the child's performance on the general articulation test and the Iowa Pressure Articulation Test. Attention should be given to eliminating hypernasality and nasal emission of consonants, especially /s/, /k/, /ʃ/, /z/, and /g/. Activating tongue tip, lip, and jaw movements (24, p. 430) and assuring an adequate mouth opening (16, p. 701) are necessary to improve articulation. For some children lip, tongue, back of the tongue, and soft palate exercises are suggested (5). A wider mouth opening on all sounds and exercise alternating open vowels such as /ɑ/ with nasal sounds helps improve movement in velar paralysis (16, p. 701). When indicated attention should be given to lowering the dorsum of the tongue especially if it is high riding (1). The speech clinician should help a child with a resonance problem develop normal activity of lips, tongue, and jaw when necessary.

Goal 2. Developing Adequate Oral Breath Pressure and Oral Air Flow

Children with velopharyngeal insufficiency need adequate oral breath pressure and oral air flow. Oral breath pressure should be increased until the proper amount is attained to produce any misarticulated sound correctly. High pressure should be reduced if it is causing misarticulation and hypernasality. When improved velar and pharyngeal contractions result in better velopharyngeal closure the person has increased oral air flow since air is not lost through nasal emission. Audible nasal emission of air during speaking should be eliminated (24, p. 430).

There is controversy concerning the use of blowing exercises in cases of velopharyngeal insufficiency. We are presenting both points of view since we feel the clinician should select remedial procedures according to the apparent needs of a child. The arguments against the use of routine blowing exercises are (11): (1) attention should be centered on correct mandible and tongue positions instead of velopharyngeal closure; (2) movements used in blowing are different from those used in speaking; (3) undesirable accessory movements, such as constriction of the nares and other facial grimaces, sometimes come about as a result of blowing exercises; (4) blowing exercises result in a misuse of breath pressure; (5) blowing exercises may result in failure and frustration. Calnan and Renfrew (6) found practice in blowing brings into play mechanisms that are useless in speech, and they concluded success in blowing activities may lead both the patient and clinician into a false hope that speech will vicariously improve. McWilliams and Bradley (14) felt the act of blowing involves a different pattern of physiological responses than those required in connected speech. Shelton, Hahn, and Morris (22, p. 257) stated we have no specific evidence to indicate motor exercises are valuable in increasing velopharyngeal competence or that exercise of palatal structures helps accomplish good and automatic articulation.

On the other hand, blowing exercises may be indicated in the treatment of hypernasality for the following reasons (11): (1) they are sometimes considered to be useful in increasing mobility of the velopharyngeal structures; (2) a nonspeech activity such as blowing exercises may motivate a person who is emotionally disturbed about his speech and resists training.

Some children improve valving and articulation as a result of vocal motor exercises and pressure building activities. In cases of very short palate, exercises can be given to train the palatal and pharyngeal muscles to function more efficiently in making the sphincter-like closure needed for normal speech (26, p. 381). This is true also in cases of hypernasality following removal of adenoid. Westlake and Rutherford (27, p. 113) stated some persons can as a result of exercises involving tactile stimulation improve valving so it becomes functional. They stated exercises are ". . . worth a *good* try." Muscle training to help velopharyngeal closure is appropriate when examination evidence shows closure is possible but not being done habitually (24, p. 434). Shelton (21) stated individuals who are inconsistent in closure during speech are usually capable of learning normal speech. He felt teaching speech skills utilizing auditory, visual, and tactile feedback should be effective for this type of person. He also stated careful study should be made of the effectiveness of exercise in increasing the range of motion of the closure mechanism. Yules and Chase (30) stated some patients with minimal velopharyngeal dysfunction may benefit from special exercises if cinefluorography demonstrates good "knee action" of the soft palate, if there is at least 2-mm posterior pharyngeal wall movement, and when nasal air escape is less than 200 cc per 12 sec. These exercises include methods for teaching the voluntary contraction of the pharyngeal wall and elevation of the soft palate. Yules and Chase prefer the use of electrical stimulation to teach voluntary contraction although other types of stimulation are effective. These include visual observation in a mirror of attempts to control velar movement and pharyngeal wall contraction. A dual channel instrument with one microphone at the nares and the other at the mouth to indicate nasal and oral resonance can be used. A meter on the instrument shows the emphasis of air flow.*

Yules and Chase (29) measured the ascent rate of the soft palate in 94 cleft palate patients, 25 velopharyngeal incompetent patients, and 36 normal subjects by the cineradiographic method. Most of the subjects were under 19 years of age. The rate of ascent in good velopharyngeal closure for the normal group was 65 mm per sec. In contrast the velopharyngeal incompetent group had an ascent rate of 38 mm per sec, while the cleft palate group was the slowest with 26 mm per sec ascent rate.

Massengill et al. (15) studied 13 cleft palate subjects aged 8 to 18 years. None of them demonstrated velopharyngeal closure when studied by cinefluorography. They investigated the effect of blowing, sucking, and swallowing exercises upon velopharyngeal closure. The subjects were divided into three groups with one group practicing blowing exercises on a manometer or with a blowing device. A second group practiced sucking exercises such as sucking through a straw or with a meter to indicate amount of pressure. The third group practiced swallowing exercises which consisted of placing the index finger on the neck in the area of the thyroid cartilage to feel neck movement during swallowing. The subjects were instructed to stop momentarily as they began to swallow and then to continue swallowing. In this way the length of the swallow was gradually increased in time. All subjects performed their specific exercises for a 20-min period each morning and each afternoon for 27 consecutive days. All subjects received intensive articulation therapy. Analysis of cinefluorographic films before and after this regime for the three groups were made on /i/ and /u/. Significantly smaller velopharyngeal closures were shown only for the group which had swallowing exercises.

Exercises

For the clinician who wishes to use exercises designed to develop adequate oral breath pressure and oral air flow, the following program is suggested. This program is based on the assumption that some children, especially those with marginal insufficiency, can benefit from a program of exercises. It is further assumed that these exercises will increase action in the velopharyngeal area, resulting in a decrease in the size of the opening. A reduction of nasal emission of sounds and hypernasality would be the dividend. Direct blowing exercises should be avoided unless the exercise is one that can accompany speech.

1. Increase the activity of the mouth, tongue, and jaw. If abnormal jaw movements and tongue movements are present the child should be taught correct jaw movements and tongue positioning. The exercises should be

* Vega Speech-O-Meter, Vega Electronics Corporation, Santa Clara, California 95050.

accompanied by vowels, words, and connected speech. Vigorous speech mechanism exercises and practice on nonsense syllables, words, and sentences using voiceless fricative consonants (/s/, /ʃ/, /f/, and /θ/) and stop-plosive consonants (/p/, /b/, /t/, /d/, /k/, and /g/) are suggested in order to improve the action of the velopharyngeal mechanism (7, pp. 224–225).

2. Reduce oral breath pressure on fricatives and stop consonants. Children with velopharyngeal insufficiency often distort articulatory movements and have nasal emission because they characteristically build up too much pressure on stop consonants or fricatives. Developing gentle stop consonants reduces the apparent nasality and air noises in velar paralysis (16, p. 701). Teaching children to use less air pressure on stop consonants or fricatives by loose contacts of the articulators allows more oral air flow; at the same time the use of larger jaw movements may facilitate better articulation and quality (2). For example, a technique using a repetitive /bɑ/, /bɑ/, /bɑ/, or /tu/, /tu/, /tu/ emphasizing easy pressure buildup and a gentle release of the /ɑ/ and /u/ sounds may be useful.

3. Develop the visual sense of palatal movement. Have the child observe the clinician's palatal movement in a mirror (24, p. 435). Next have the child watch as he himself voluntarily elevates the soft palate and contacts the pharyngeal wall (30). Then the child can be taught the kinesthetic sensations of pharyngeal wall contraction. These exercises should be accompanied by speech.

4. Speed up palatal ascent rate. We feel it may be possible to speed up the rate of palatal ascent in a child with velopharyngeal incompetence through vocal motor exercises and pressure-building activities. In this way we may obtain better closure for speech and thus decrease hypernasality and nasal emission. Improved articulation and resonance should result.

5. Froeschels' pushing exercises may be useful (4, p. 673). These are described in Chapter 5. They improve velopharyngeal closure and help speed up the ascent rate of the soft palate.

6. Eliminate the glottal stop. A glottal stop may be substituted for various pressure sounds by children with velopharyngeal insufficiency. These children substitute a buildup of pressure at the level of the glottis for a buildup of pressure within the oral cavity to produce pressure sounds. The speech clinician can have the child listen through a stethoscope with the bell of the stethoscope near the clinician's larynx; the clinician then demonstrates the difference between a glottal stop and the correct production of the sound. Then the child listens in a similar fashion to his own production of glottal stops. He continues to listen as the glottal stops are eliminated and he learns good production of pressure sounds (3).

7. Practice the swallowing exercises used in the Massengill *et al.* study (15) described earlier in this chapter.

Goal 3. Improving Voice Quality

Improving voice quality is based on careful listening training. The child is then ready for instruction in reducing or eliminating hypernasality. Negative practice is useful in eliminating hypernasality and nasal emission.

Listening Training

The correction of articulation errors improves voice quality but most children need specific work to reduce hypernasality and nasal emission. Listening training teaches a child the differences between hypernasal quality and normal quality. Williamson (28) found in 84 cases, with few exceptions, few if any velopharyngeal closure exercises are necessary if a person with hypernasality is given a remedial program stressing the auditory aspects of good voice. Many children with hypernasality interpret their own voice quality as sounding the same as the normal voices they hear. Therefore, they must be taught to hear the difference between a non-nasal and a nasal voice (18, p. 173; 19). It is necessary in cases of velar paralysis to develop the ability to listen carefully to voice and speech in order to produce the most intelligible communication possible (16, p. 701).

We have found improvement of quality is based upon thorough listening training following the general outline in Chapter 4. Listening training is designed to decrease hypernasality as well as reduce the emission of sounds through the nose. Listening training follows the three major steps: (1) awareness of the difference in others, (2) gross discrimination of differences in others, and (3) fine discrimination of differences in others. In all steps the speech clinician is the performer while the child is the listener and judge. The clinician uses the child's most hypernasal phonemes for listening training. These procedures teach the child to listen and to make judgments about voice quality in the clinician's speech.

The listening training program for hypernasal voice begins with awareness of the difference. For example the clinician uses pairs of sounds or words, saying one of the pair with hypernasal quality and the other with normal quality. The child signals the presence of the defective aspect by raising his hand or dropping a bead in a box when he hears the hypernasal quality. Many similar techniques of interest to the child can be devised to teach awareness of the defective quality as the clinician speaks sounds, syllables, words, or sentences using the undesirable voice on some of the items. In gross discrimination two levels, excessive hypernasality and normal quality, are presented for the child to judge differences. Pairs of sounds using the two vocal parameters are spoken by the clinician while the child judges which is which. Fine discrimination of differences calls for even more careful listening and judging by the child. He is required to make judgments of the extent of defectiveness of quality in the clinician's speech.

Usually three levels are selected representing excessive hypernasality, moderate hypernasality, and normal quality. For example the clinician produces a series of three /ɑ/ sounds with the three degrees of voice quality. The child can indicate his judgment by placing a bead or block in one of three designated boxes or by simply giving verbal indication of recognition of variations. The differences at first can be quite great but as listening training proceeds the differences are decreased until expert listening by the child is required.

Reduction or Elimination of Hypernasality

After listening training has developed the child's ability to discriminate between varying amounts of hypernasality in the clinician's voice, the child is ready to work directly on improving the quality of his own voice. The clinician stimulates the child by saying the correct sound or word several times. Then he asks the child to imitate him. Improvement of quality is many times dependent on developing new kinesthetic patterns of correct tongue placement and wider mouth opening. If habitual excessive loudness makes the voice more nasal it is desirable to decrease the loudness.

Van Riper and Irwin (25, pp. 248–251) stated reducing the assimilation effect of nasal sounds and increasing the amount of non-nasal phonation in general is essential. They recommended selecting a phoneme that is excessively nasal and reducing the nasality on that one phoneme. This greatly increases the amount of non-nasal phonation in general. They reported that their most successful cases have been those who were taught normal production of one or two of the most nasalized vowels and then fixing and stabilizing these phonemes.

Negative Practice

Negative practice can be used to reinforce and strengthen the use of improved resonance. For example to reduce nasal emission the child is asked to produce a sound with nasal emission immediately followed by production of the sound without nasal emission. Negative practice usually begins by using isolated sounds and progresses to syllables, words, and finally sentences. A child with velopharyngeal insufficiency especially needs negative practice during all aspects of his program. This type of practice allows the child to gain control over new habits and leads to eventual habituation.

Improving Voice Quality in Hyponasality

Voice therapy is essential when hyponasality is present on a functional basis. It may also be indicated following operations for removal of nasal obstructions. In some cases the person's auditory feedback is such that he continues to use hyponasal speech even though the nasal passage is open. The basic procedures for improving voice quality in hypernasality can be modified to apply to children with hyponasal voice quality. The listening training procedures remain the same with the speech clinician using a hyponasal voice. The speech clinician must teach the child how to produce nasal sounds and when they should be used. A child can be taught to hum a prolonged /m/ and then taught to produce the /n/ and /ŋ/; after these have been learned in isolation the child is ready to practice them in syllables, words, and then sentences in free conversation (4, p. 686). Increasing the phonation time on /m/, /n/, and /ŋ/ in connected speech decreases the impression of hyponasality (20).

An unusual combination of hypernasality and hyponasality sometimes occurs (4, p. 687; 17, p. 59; 26, p. 389). Some persons may have a partial obstruction in the nasal passages interfering with production of normal nasal sounds /m/, /n/, and /ŋ/, but strangely they may nasalize some vowels or consonants. The program for this problem, according to West and Ansberry (26, p. 389), includes the following: (1) explain the causes of both types of resonance problems, (2) administer a thorough program of listening training, (3) practice for control of velopharyngeal closure, (4) teach adequate nasalization on /m/, /n/, and /ŋ/, and (5) improve articulation ability especially in connected speech.

Goal 4. Eliminating Facial Grimaces and Nares Constriction

A child with velopharyngeal insufficiency may unconsciously constrict his nares in an effort to prevent nasal emission of sound. He may also have associated facial grimaces. Improving velopharyngeal closure and articulation may eliminate nares constriction and facial grimaces since they are no longer necessary. However, it may be necessary to work directly on eliminating these habits if they have become a firmly fixed part of the speaking pattern. It can be done by bringing their use to the conscious level by using negative practice and eventually eliminating them through mirror work (24, p. 441).

Goal 5. Modifying or Eliminating Vocal Abuse and Establishing Balanced Muscular Tonus

The clinician should listen for hoarseness or any other signs of developing vocal cord difficulties since children with velopharyngeal insufficiency may have vocal cord abnormalities. McDonald and Baker (11) stated vocal cord hyperemia and hyperplasia are characteristic of many persons with cleft palate. McWilliams, Bluestone, and Musgrave (13) found most of a group of children with cleft palates with hoarse voices had vocal nodules or vocal cord changes. The speech clinician should note any vocal abuse, analyze it carefully, and proceed with a program for its elimination or modification. Our program for eliminating or modifying vocal abuse described in Chapter 5 can be used for children with velopharyngeal insufficiency.

Children with velopharyngeal insufficiency may require attention to balanced muscular tonus. They are likely to develop abnormal muscular tensions when they attempt to speak clearly. Luse, Heisse, and Foley (10) reported on three patients with repaired cleft palates whose speech had marked cleft palate quality. Two of them had vocal cord pathology, one, aged 10 years, had vocal nodules and the other, aged 21, had contact ulcers. The vocal cord pathologies and the poor voice quality were felt to be due to pharyngeal and laryngeal tension. Initial x-ray lateral head plates showed a retracted tongue and a constricted pharyngeal wall. Following therapy procedures which emphasized release of tension in the laryngeal and pharyngeal areas, the vocal pathologies were no longer present and the voice quality was reported to be close to normal in all three patients. At this point x-ray lateral head plates showed the ball of the tongue tended to move away from the pharyngeal wall and the pharyngeal airway assumed a more normal appearance for phonation. When any unusual tensions are present in children with velopharyngeal insufficiences our procedures for achieving balanced muscular tonus described in Chapter 5 can be incorporated into the program. The clinician may need to make particular use of the exercises for reducing hyperfunction in laryngeal and pharyngeal areas. All efforts should be made to prevent the development of muscular tensions as the child strives to improve articulation and to establish adequate oral breath pressure.

Goal 6. Establishing Adequate Use of Loudness, Pitch, and Speaking Rate

During the examination, evaluations of a child's use of loudness, pitch, and speaking rate were made. Any significant deviations from normal should receive attention. If the voice is too loud or too soft the loudness training program described in Chapter 5 can be followed. Children with pitch and rate deviations can receive programs described in the same chapter for appropriate modification. Changes in loudness, pitch, or rate should not be made unless they deviate from normal. The speech clinician can compare these voice parameters in a particular child with norms or standards and make appropriate changes.

Children with resonance problems need carefully programmed voice therapy. Correctly balanced oral and nasal resonance is based upon improving articulation and speech intelligibility. Special attention should be given to listening training in the programs to reduce or eliminate hypernasality and hyponasality. Eliminating facial grimaces and nares constriction results in cosmetic improvement. Modifying or eliminating vocal abuse and establishing balanced muscular tonus are necessary for improving the quality of the laryngeal tone. Adequate use of loudness, appropriate pitch, and suitable rate of speaking are basic to improved resonance. Using proper oral breath pressure and oral air flow improves both voice quality and articulation. Special therapeutic exercises may improve resonance in selected children. A comprehensive voice therapy program enables a child to use good resonance with adequate speech intelligibility.

REFERENCES

1. Adler, S. Some techniques for treating the hypernasal voice. *J. Speech Hearing Dis.*, **25**, 1960, 300–302.
2. Anonymous. Clinical suggestions. *W. Mich. Univ. J. Speech Ther.*, **1**, 1964, 6.
3. Anonymous. Helpful hints. *W. Mich. Univ. J. Speech Ther.*, **1**, 1964, 6–7.
4. Arnold, G. E. Physiology and pathology of speech and language. In R. Luchsinger and G. E. Arnold. *Voice—speech—language. Clinical communicology: Its physiology and pathology*. Belmont: Wadsworth Publishing Company, 1965.
5. Buck, M., and Harrington, R. Organized speech therapy for cleft palate rehabilitation. *J. Speech Hearing Dis.*, **14**, 1949, 43–52.
6. Calnan, J., and Renfrew, C. E. Blowing tests and speech. *Brit. J. Plast. Surg.*, **13**, 1961, 340–346.
7. Curtis, J. F. Disorders of voice. In W. Johnson and D. Moeller (Editors), *Speech handicapped school children*. Ed. 3. New York: Harper and Row, 1967.
8. Fletcher, S. G. Hypernasal voice as an indication of regional growth and developmental disturbances. *Logos*, **3**, 1960, 3–12.
9. Glenn, J. W., and Kleiner, N. Speaker identification based on nasal phonation. *J. Acoust. Soc. Amer.*, **43**, 1968, 368–371.
10. Luse, E., Heisse, J., and Foley, J. The vocal approach in the correction of cleft palate speech. *Folia Phoniat. (Basel)*, **16**, 1964, 123–129.
11. McDonald, E. T., and Baker, H. K. Cleft palate speech: An integration of research and clinical observation. *J. Speech Hearing Dis.*, **16**, 1951, 9–20.
12. McWilliams, B. J. Some factors in the intelligibility of cleft palate speech. *J. Speech Hearing Dis.*, **19**, 1954, 524–527.
13. McWilliams, B. J., Bluestone, C. D., and Musgrave, R. D. Diagnostic implications of vocal cord nodules in children with cleft palate. *Laryngoscope*, **79**, 1969, 2072–2080.
14. McWilliams, B. J., and Bradley, D. P. Ratings of velopharyngeal closure during blowing and speech. *Cleft Palate J.*, **2**, 1965, 46–55.
15. Massengill, R., Jr., Quinn, G. W., Pickrell, K. L., and Levinson, C. Therapeutic exercise and velopharyngeal gap. *Cleft Palate J.*, **5**, 1968, 44–47.
16. Moore, G. P. Voice disorders associated with organic abnormalities. In L. E. Travis (Editor), *Handbook of speech pathology*. New York: Appleton-Century-Crofts, Inc., 1957.
17. Murphy, A. T. *Functional voice disorders*. Englewood Cliffs: Prentice-Hall, Inc., 1964.
18. Mysak, E. D. Phonatory and resonatory problems. In R. W. Rieber and R. S. Brubaker (Editors), *Speech pathology. An international study of the science*. Philadelphia: J. B. Lippincott Company, 1966.
19. Porterfield, H. W., Trabue, J. C., Terry, J. L., and Stimpert, R. D. Hypernasality in non-cleft palate patients. *J. Plast. Reconstr. Surg.*, **37**, 1966, 216–220.
20. Scholl, H. M. A holistic approach to the teaching of voice improvement. *Speech Teacher*, **10**, 1961, 200–205.
21. Shelton, R. L., Jr. Therapeutic exercise and speech pathology. *Asha*, **5**, 1963, 855–859.
22. Shelton, R. L., Jr., Hahn, E., and Morris, H. L. Diagnosis and therapy. In D. C. Spriestersbach and D. Sherman (Editors), *Cleft palate and communication*. New York: Academic Press, 1968.

23. Tobias, J. V. Relative occurrence of phonemes in American English. *J. Acoust. Soc. Amer.*, **31**, 1959, 631.
24. Van Riper, C. *Speech correction. Principles and methods*. Ed. 4. Englewood Cliffs: Prentice-Hall, Inc., 1963.
25. Van Riper, C., and Irwin, J. V. *Voice and articulation*. Englewood Cliffs: Prentice-Hall, Inc., 1958.
26. West, R. W., and Ansberry, M. *The rehabilitation of speech*. Ed. 4. New York: Harper and Row, 1968.
27. Westlake, H., and Rutherford, D. *Cleft palate*. Englewood Cliffs: Prentice-Hall, Inc., 1966.
28. Williamson, A. B. Diagnosis and treatment of 84 cases of nasality. *Quart. J. Speech*, **30**, 1944, 471–479.
29. Yules, R. B., and Chase, R. A. Quantitative ciné evaluation of palates and pharyngeal wall mobility in normal palates, in cleft palates, and in velopharyngeal incompetency. *J. Plast. Reconstr. Surg.*, **41**, 1968, 124–128.
30. Yules, R. B., and Chase, R. A. A training method for reduction of hypernasality in speech. *J. Plast. Reconstr. Surg.*, **43**, 1969, 180–185.

7

VOICE PROBLEMS OF CHILDREN
WITH HEARING LOSSES

Many children with hearing losses have voice problems. Silverman and Davis (21, p. 427) indicated voice problems appear in children with hearing losses for speech of 56 dB (ISO, 1964) and greater. Fuller (9, pp. 208–209) stated voice quality is affected in children with flat audiograms with threshold levels greater than 50 dB, or in children with losses 40 dB or greater in the low frequencies with greater loss in the high frequencies. Irwin (13, p. 255) reported inadequate voice quality was noted in 22 % of a group of 284 children referred to otological clinics.

Early voice training not only helps prevent the development of voice problems but also insures a more adequate voice for effective speech communication (27). The clinician should listen carefully for the natural quality and pitch of very young hearing-impaired children's voices as they babble and vocalize during play; the child should be helped to maintain this pleasant voice quality, avoiding the development of a nasal or strained voice (16).

The program of voice therapy presented in this chapter is designed for use by a school or clinic speech clinician in handling voice problems of hearing-impaired children enrolled in a regular classroom. Speech clinicians in regular schools and in speech clinics are concerned principally with the voices of children with *aided* hearing of approximately 45 dB (ISO, 1964) or better. However, the unaided hearing loss may vary considerably and in some cases may be as great as 85 dB (ISO, 1964, average of 500, 1000, 2000 Hz). Some children with severe losses have had extensive early training and are being educated in regular classrooms. Pollack (18, p. 165) stated, "We are now facing a new generation of limited hearing children. They have been diagnosed in early infancy, fitted with powerful binaural hearing aids, bathed in sound and stimulated by an intensive auditory approach during the critical period for learning speech and language." The speech clinician must be prepared for voice therapy with this "new generation" because, as Pollack (18, pp. 157–165) indicated, many of them can attend school with normal hearing children. These children may be included in the case load of a school speech clinician.

Medical and Audiological Examinations

The speech clinician must exercise the same care in obtaining medical clearance before initiating voice therapy for a hearing-impaired child as for a child with normal hearing. It is assumed children have received the necessary otological attention before the speech clinician sees them. Irwin (13, p. 255) stated problems of voice quality in hearing-impaired children often appear to be related to pathologies of the nose, throat, or ear. Streng *et al.* (22, p. 228) indicated breathy, harsh, or hypernasal voices found in children with hearing losses are not necessarily related to the loss. The possibility of vocal pathology in children with impaired hearing must be considered. For example, Arnold (1, p. 637) stated children with hearing impairments may increase their vocal intensity in order to hear themselves better and they may as a result develop vocal nodules. Medical consultation, especially regarding laryngeal dysfunction and velopharyngeal insufficiency, is indicated. Voice therapy may be coordinated with recommended medical procedures or postponed until the results of these procedures can be determined.

The results of audiological evaluations should be available to the speech clinician. He is particularly interested in the child's hearing ability without a hearing aid and in a detailed analysis of the improvements resulting from hearing aid use. The report should include speech reception thresholds and speech discrimination scores without and with a hearing aid.

Examination Procedures by the Speech Clinician

Prior to initiating voice therapy for a child with a hearing loss, his voice should be evaluated carefully to determine the areas needing attention. The speech clinician should be on the alert for voice problems typically found in hearing-impaired children. These problems include undesirable resonance, improper use of pitch, inappropriate loudness, defective laryngeal tone, and inadequate rate. Typical resonance problems are hypernasality, hyponasality, and a hollow muffled quality usually referred to as cul-de-sac resonance. Pitch may be too high, too low, and monotonous. Vocal intensity may be too soft or too loud. Laryngeal dysfunction may be present causing the voice to sound breathy, harsh, or hoarse. The rate of speaking may be slow and monotonous.

The examination procedures described in Chapter 3 for use with normal hearing children can be used or adapted to hearing-impaired children. Ratings to assess vocal parameters should be made at the beginning of training to establish baselines and then repeated periodically to chart progress. All items of the group play observation chart (Fig. 17) give useful preliminary information. The use of the general voice profile (Fig. 18) is essential; any items not rated normal should be evaluated in more detail.

For example, if a child has improper use of pitch, his habitual pitch level should be determined and compared with norms in Tables 2 and 3. It may be necessary to evaluate the child's use of loudness carefully. If resonance appears to be a problem, the resonance profile (Fig. 19) should be completed. Children with hypernasal voices should be given the Iowa Pressure Articulation Test and appropriate oral and nasal air flow measures discussed in Chapter 3. If vocal abuse is noted, it should be carefully evaluated using the vocal abuse rating chart (Fig. 21).

Voice Therapy

With appropriate modifications our general programs of voice therapy for children with normal hearing can be used for hearing-impaired children enrolled in regular classrooms. The modifications depend mainly upon the child's aided hearing. We will suggest some of the appropriate modifications and will include supplementary exercises from programs for deaf children. We recommend the following general principles for voice therapy in the presence of a hearing loss: (1) full use should be made of the auditory pathway; (2) the voice therapy program must always be coordinated closely with the child's overall program, including auditory training, lip reading, improvement of articulation, vocabulary building, and speech conservation; (3) the auditory approach should be supplemented by visual stimuli and training in the use of kinesthetic and tactile cues.

Our program of voice therapy for hearing-impaired children makes full use of the auditory pathway using our listening training program. This program should be based on the child's previous auditory training and combined with his current auditory training program. According to Sanders (20, p. 205), "Auditory training constitutes a systematic procedure designed to increase the amount of information that a person's hearing contributes to his total perception." Auditory training is an integral part of the program for a child with a hearing loss, and it ranges all the way from gross discrimination of noises to fine discrimination of speech sounds.

Although we place primary emphasis on an auditory approach, we recommend supplementing it with visual stimulation and with kinesthetic and tactile cues. Pollack (18, p. 19) advocated a primarily auditory approach to teaching very young children; then when the listening function has been established she recommended supplementing auditory cues with visual cues. According to Berg (2, p. 305) supplementation of auditory stimulation with visual and tactile aids should occur when the child is between 3 and 5 years of age. The use of tactile and kinesthetic cues, according to New (17), helps the child develop an "inner feeling," specifically in the region of the throat and neck, as to what is desirable and undesirable; this helps him control quality and pitch. The clinician signals to the child when he is producing the desired pitch, loudness, or quality. With training the child can develop the ability to supplement his auditory cues with the tactile and kinesthetic sensations of the desired voice productions. Froeschels (7; 8) recommended the use of his chewing method, described in Chapter 5, to improve the voices of hard of hearing and deaf children. He felt the use of this method, with special attention to the kinesthesia of chewing and of improved voice quality, helps to replace unusual voice patterns with more normal patterns for these children.

Carryover and habituation may prove to be especially slow in the presence of a hearing impairment (15). The habituation procedures described in Chapter 4 should be followed. Habituation, especially in children with hearing impairments, requires much time, patience, and perseverance on the part of the speech clinician, the child, his family, and his teachers.

Goals of Voice Therapy

The goals of voice therapy for children with a voice problem in the presence of a hearing loss are: (1) balanced resonance, without excessive hypernasality, hyponasality, or the cul-de-sac effect; (2) proper habitual pitch level with appropriate expressive pitch variations; (3) control of loudness; (4) a clear laryngeal tone free from hypertension and hypotension; (5) correct rate and rhythm of speaking; (6) elimination or modification of vocal abuse.

Each goal is attained by proceeding through the three basic procedures of voice therapy: listening training, teaching correct voice use, and habituation of correct voice use. The most defective aspect of voice is selected to begin concentrated listening training. However, with most children we work on several aspects of defective voice simultaneously. For example, because of the close interrelationship of loudness and pitch, these are often given simultaneous attention. Inappropriate use of rate may also be included in a simultaneous approach.

Goal 1. Resonance

The resonance problem in a child with a hearing loss may be hypernasality, hyponasality, or the hollow muffled quality typical of cul-de-sac resonance. The program for teaching the child with a hearing loss to use proper resonance begins with the basic listening training program. This program, following the procedures described in Chapters 4 and 6, includes (1) making the child aware of resonance differences in others, (2) gross discrimination of resonance differences in others, and (3) fine discrimination of differences in others. Then the listening training program is applied to the child's own voice. He is made aware of resonance defects in himself, followed by gross and fine discrimination of differences of resonance in his own voice. Upon completion of these procedures he is then ready to learn to control proper resonance and eventually use the new resonance habitually.

The problem of hypernasality will be used to illustrate the methods of improving resonance. First, the clinician produces vowels, words, and phrases with excessive hypernasality on some productions and normal resonance on others. The child indicates when he hears the hypernasal production. Initially amplification with an auditory trainer is useful to make sure the child receives a strong signal. Soon, however, the child should use his own hearing aid. Second, the clinician produces excessively hypernasal productions and normal productions requiring the child to discriminate between the two by indicating which is which. Third, the clinician randomly produces sounds with varying degrees of resonance from severely hypernasal through moderate and mild hypernasality to normal resonance for the child to discriminate.

When the child becomes proficient in discrimination of hypernasality in others he is ready to apply his learning to himself. The clinician prepares recordings of the child's voice. The child listens to these recordings of his own productions following the pattern used in discriminating hypernasality in the clinician's voice. Now he must become aware of excessively hypernasal productions in his recordings, identifying only the very worst ones. Next he listens to his recordings, identifying the excessively hypernasal productions and those with normal resonance. Then he discriminates very fine differences in his own productions ranging from excessively hypernasal to normal.

Now the child is an expert in identifying and discriminating hypernasality of varying degrees and normal resonance in both others and himself. He is ready to begin control of resonance in himself. The recordings of the child are used as models of production. The child listens to these recordings doing negative practice of varying degrees of hypernasality contrasted with his productions of normal resonance. In this way the child obtains voluntary control of resonance and is able to reduce or eliminate hypernasality. With appropriate adaptations this general program is used for hyponasality and the cul-de-sac effect.

Many additional techniques should be used with the hearing-impaired child to help him learn better use of resonance. The use of the Vega Speech-O-Meter* helps the child discriminate between hypernasal, hyponasal, and normal resonance and is an aid in the production of improved resonance. The child should be taught the kinesthetic and tactile sensations that signal to him the adequate use of resonance. Have the child learn tactile sensations by placing his fingers lightly on the clinician's nose, comparing the presence of vibrations during hypernasal speech with the absence of vibrations during non-nasal speech. Then have the child do the same on himself. A series of vowels with /m/, /n/, and /ŋ/ can be used, for example, /u-n/, /ɑ-n/, /o-n/, /i-n/.

* Vega Speech-O-Meter, Vega Electronics Corporation, Santa Clara, California 95050.

The following exercises were recommended by Haycock (11, pp. 100–102), and are to be performed with the child observing himself in a mirror.

1. Instruct the child to open his mouth, lower the back of the tongue and place the tongue tip firmly behind the lower incisors. Holding this tongue position, have the child breathe in and out strongly several times.

2. Have the child close his lips, inhale through the nose, then open the mouth for the exhalation. While he does this the tongue should be low in the mouth and the throat relaxed.

3. With his mouth wide open, have the child inhale through the nose and exhale through his mouth.

4. Have the child phonate /ŋ-ɑ/ several times, noting the visual, auditory, kinesthetic, and tactile differences between them.

5. Have the child say a series of vowel sounds followed by /ŋ/, for example /u-o-ɑ-i-ŋ/, prolonging the /ŋ/. Have the child do the same exercise followed by /m/ and then by /n/.

The hollow cul-de-sac resonance quality often heard in individuals with hearing losses is sometimes prevented by early hearing aid use and early attention to voice. Since it is usually associated with hypernasal or hyponasal speech, attention to proper nasal resonance may result in a modification of the cul-de-sac resonance. However, in some children it requires direct attention through a program based on listening training and supplemented by special techniques. Boone (4) felt cul-de-sac quality is due to a focus of resonance in the pharyngeal area related to retraction of the tongue toward the pharyngeal wall. He recommended the following exercise designed to keep the tongue low in the mouth with the tongue tip forward and to increase oral resonance. Have the child start with a whispered repetitive /tɑ/, /tɑ/, /tɑ/, /tɑ/ and then whisper /dɑ/, /sɑ/, and /zɑ/ in the same way. The exercise is repeated using voice. These alveolar tongue-tip sounds should be practiced in rapid drill for about 5 min four or five times daily. Boone also used the consonants /w/, /p/, /b/, /f/, /v/, /θ/, /ð/, and /l/ combined with vowels having a high oral focus, such as /i/, /ɪ/. /e/, /ɛ/, and /æ/.

Goal 2. Pitch

The habitual pitch level of a child with a hearing loss should be checked periodically and compared with norms for his age to make sure the high pitch of childhood does not persist as he matures. Although individuals vary, young hearing-impaired children generally use a fundamental frequency within the normal range. For example, Meckfessel (14) found deaf boys 7 and 8 years of age had a mean fundamental frequency of 292 Hz and normal hearing boys 289 Hz. Also, Ermovick (6) found the mean fundamental frequency of deaf girls the same age was 235 Hz and of normal hearing girls 245 Hz. All these figures fall within the normal limits of our pitch tables (Tables 2 and 3). However, a group of deaf males 17 and 18 years of age had a mean fundamental frequency of 184 Hz and the normal hearing group 130 Hz (14), a difference of one-half octave which is significant. The normal hearing group is comparable to our norms (Table 2) while the mean of the deaf boys is definitely higher than our acceptable limits. The situation is a little different for girls of this age. No statistical difference was found between the mean fundamental frequencies of 256 Hz for the deaf girls and 230 Hz for normal hearing girls (6). However, while the figure for hearing girls is within our acceptable limits (Table 3) the mean for deaf girls is slightly above our upper limit. Boone (4), commenting on this study, stated there was wide variation among the older deaf girls with some of them having very high pitch; these girls should be taught to use a lower habitual pitch.

The basic procedures for improvement of pitch can be built around the steps on the pitch chart (Fig. 30): "1. I know the rule about the pitch of my voice. 2. I can tell when other people use high and low voices. 3. I can hear when the pitch of my voice is wrong. 4. I can hear the correct pitch in my voice. 5. I know the places where I use the wrong pitch. 6. I know the places where I use the correct pitch. 7. I can talk with the correct pitch *some* of the time. 8. I can talk with the correct pitch *most* of the time. 9. I can talk with the correct pitch *all* the time." If any of these steps prove to be especially difficult for a child with a hearing loss, the clinician can take emphasis off the chart temporarily until the child has mastered the difficult steps.

The clinician should apply the basic listening training program to pitch. This would follow the pattern of learning to identify the undesirable pitch in others, and then proceeding to gross discrimination and fine discrimination of pitch differences in others. For example, a tape recorder can be used to establish better pitch discrimination. The clinician first records his own voice using a high pitch and then a very low pitch asking the child to make gross discriminations. The clinician then uses three different levels, high, middle, and low, with the middle tone at the child's normal speaking level. The child makes fine discriminations between these three levels. The pitch differences between the tones can be reduced for discriminating extremely small differences. Then the clinician uses recordings of the child to teach awareness of undesirable pitch in his own voice. The child listens to his recordings to identify undesirable pitch as well as the desired pitch level. This first is done through gross discrimination of two widely different levels of pitch such as very high and normal. The training proceeds to the final step of listening training—fine discrimination of three or more levels of pitch, very high, high, normal, and low. The singing voice can be used in a similar manner (19). The speech clinician should check with the classroom and music teachers to coordinate training in pitch discrimination with other discrimination training the child is receiving.

Some hard of hearing children may be able to proceed through the stages of listening training with only slightly more practice than children with normal hearing. For others special methods of developing pitch discrimination may be needed. If the child initially is unable to distinguish pitch differences in the clinician's voice, a piano, musical instrument, toy horn, or toy xylophone may be used to present widely different tones for discrimination. The clinician then proceeds to discrimination of voice. The training can be made more interesting by varying the child's responses as well as the stimuli. The child is asked to lift his hands above his head for a high tone, touch his shoulders for a medium tone, and stoop toward the floor for a low tone (22, p. 214). The head, waist, or knees could be touched for other intermediate tones. If stair steps are available in the therapy room, the child can climb to the top step when he hears a high tone and return to lower steps and the floor for intermediate and low tones. As the child improves in pitch discrimination the clinician can read or tell stories, using a variety of pitch for different characters (22, p. 214).

Visual aids can be helpful in developing pitch discrimination. Lights of different colors can be flashed when different pitches are presented (22, p. 322). When working with young children appropriate mechanical toys can be activated when various pitch levels are presented, for example, a bird for high pitch, a clown for medium pitch, and a dancing bear for low pitch. An older child can view an oscilloscope or the VU meter of a pitch meter to aid him in identifying various pitches produced by the clinician.

When the child is ready to produce the desired pitch level the program for teaching correct pitch described in Chapter 5 should be followed. Additional techniques may be necessary for the hearing-impaired child. The following procedures for developing control of pitch are based on Streng et al. (22, p. 230): (1) the child imitates the clinician as he hums gliding up and down the scale; (2) the clinician hums middle C, B, or B flat below middle C. The child feels the vibrations in the clinician's face and throat and then imitates these notes; (3) the child imitates specific notes produced by the clinician using tactile and kinesthetic cues; (4) the clinician hums /m/ at the child's optimum pitch while the child says the following syllables at this pitch: /m/-/ɑ/, /m/-/ɑ/, /mɑ/; /m/-/ɔ/, /m/-/ɔ/, /mɔ/; /m/-/o/, /m/-/o/, /mo/; the child then hums one octave higher and produces these syllables at this pitch; the child does the same thing one-half octave higher than his optimum pitch; (5) the child speaks short sentences in a monotone at the correct pitch level; (6) the child then uses normal variations of pitch while saying these sentences; (7) the child uses variations of pitch while telling stories and participating in dramatic sketches.

Synchronous reading may be helpful (10, pp. 221–222; 3, p. 467; 25). The clinician reads in unison with the child on a binaural trainer. The intensity of the clinician's voice is gradually increased until the child hears only the clinician's voice. He then may follow the pitch variations he hears. This can be done to help obtain correct pitch level, inflections, and rhythm. This should be done carefully to be sure the child is actually following the pitch variations he hears. Children with hearing impairments should be taught to sing at a very early age. Singing enables hearing-impaired children to maintain or to develop more suitable pitch and inflections in their speech.

Disturbed mutation can be a problem in a hearing-impaired adolescent. The methods described in Chapter 5 can be used for these young people. Engleberg (5) described the following program he used in working on a falsetto voice in a deaf female 20 years of age. Phonate while the head is extended backward. Phonate on request at a lower pitch. Phonate at the highest pitch, dropping suddenly to the lowest pitch. The sounds to be used with this technique are /ɑ/, /o/, and /i/, /mɑ/, and the word *mama*. Counting from 1 through 10 is used, paying particular attention to pitch control and avoiding forced respiration. Sessions are also devoted to improving vocal inflection, progressing from reading to general conversation.

The deflection of the needle on the VU meter of the pitch meter is particularly useful in indicating to the hard of hearing adolescent when his pitch level is appropriate and when he is making adequate use of pitch inflections. This aids the adolescent in exploring vocal ranges and gives him a visual indication of the appropriate pitch level (4). The youth can be taught to produce the desired pitch level by checking his pitch on the pitch meter and then asking him to note the kinesthetic and tactile sensations when he produces the desired pitch. The clinician should immediately compare this with the person's old inappropriate pitch by comparing the tactile and kinesthetic sensations of the two.

Goal 3. Loudness

The modification of loudness follows the general pattern of listening training, learning to produce the desired level, and habituation. The loudness chart (Fig. 32) is appropriate for use with a hard of hearing child. If the child's voice is too soft the same chart can be used with the items reworded appropriately.

To add interest to identification and discrimination of loudness levels in the clinician's voice, pictures can be placed in the child's notebook to illustrate the different levels. These can be pictures of people speaking at different levels (Fig. 31); they can also be pictures of vehicles, machines, or animals which make different levels of noise, or they can be pictures of children engaging in activities ranging from quiet to noisy. The child can be asked to point to the appropriate picture as the clinician uses each different level of voice.

The following special techniques recommended by Streng *et al.* (22, pp. 212–213) for developing loudness control in young hearing-impaired children will be useful if loudness training presents a problem: (1) compare loud stomping with tiptoeing, loud clapping with soft clapping, and loud music with soft music; (2) play a hide and seek game as the child searches for a hidden toy; play music with the loudness regulated according to the nearness of the child to the toy; (3) the child sings or hums softly and then loudly to relate the concept of loudness or softness to his own voice; (4) teach the child to increase speech intensity in noisy surroundings and decrease it in quiet places; take him into both types of situations; we recommend calling attention to auditory, kinesthetic, and tactile cues to show him correct loudness in the presence of varying levels of background noise.

The intensity indicator of a recorder, an oscilloscope, or sound level meter can be used in teaching the child to use a desired loudness. The child watches the visual indicator as he uses different loudness levels with the clinician telling him when the loudness level is adequate. In this way the child can coordinate the visual indication with what he hears and feels as he is speaking and he can adjust his loudness level accordingly. He can be given supervised practice on different levels in different situations until he has a feeling for the level most suitable for each. Work on appropriate loudness can be incorporated into the general auditory training program and combined with procedures to improve other parameters of voice. Repeated verbal comments on appropriate loudness in various situations will be effective in helping the child correct any deficiency in the use of appropriate loudness.

Goal. 4 Laryngeal Tone

Voice therapy designed to improve resonance, pitch, and loudness adds flexibility to the voice and often has the added effect of eliminating or modifying harshness, breathiness, and hoarseness. Programs for persistent harshness or hoarseness following procedures for laryngeal dysfunction described in Chapter 5 should be used when necessary.

Special attention should be given to breathiness because it is a frequently encountered laryngeal dysfunction in children with hearing impairments. For this problem we suggest applying our complete program of listening training to breathiness. Some of the procedures described in Chapter 5 for hypofunction are useful in eliminating breathiness.

Hudgins (12) felt elimination of breathiness depends upon the ability to adjust the laryngeal muscles in proper relationship to breath pressure in forming speech sounds. The following series of exercises which he found successful in reducing breathiness in a group of profoundly deaf children with breathy voices can be used for hard of hearing children.

1. Have the child hold his breath for a reasonable period with the chest slightly inflated and the mouth open. Ask the child to pant in this position, exhaling and inhaling small puffs of air at the rate of about 2 or 3 a sec. This is designed to teach control of the breath supply by use of chest and abdominal muscles.

2. Have the child assume the inflated chest position with the mouth open and exhale a series of puffs of air between inhalations. He is to stop the breath flow between each puff of air. The child does not inhale until he has completed the series of puffs. The number of puffs must be specified, using four or six at first. Each series is followed by a rapid inhalation through the mouth. Do not allow the child to use his entire breath supply in any one series, and do not allow him to revert to the panting exercise. The speed of the pulses should approximate the rate of syllables in normal speech.

3. The next step is designed to develop normal vocal attack. At first have the child produce a tone briefly to make sure he is using the proper amount of tension in the larynx. Proper tension is present when breathiness is absent. Then have him phonate a prolonged /ɑ/. If the tone does not retain a natural quality throughout its duration, the child should be stopped and asked to start over. When he can use a good voice on /ɑ/, he is then asked to produce /u/ and /i/ in the same way.

4. Have the child phonate repetitive vowels on puffs of air, first using /ɑ/ and later proceeding to the /u/ and /i/. The child should start with a series of four or six syllables on a single breath and gradually increase the number. He should maintain good posture and proper laryngeal adjustment, avoiding breathiness on the tone. At first each series consists of a single vowel. Then he is asked to change from one vowel to another in a series, for example, /ɑ/, /u/, /i/, /u/, /i/, /ɑ/. The rate of the vowel production should correspond to normal speaking rate.

5. The basic procedure of the preceding exercise is used, but this time ask the child to alternate a loud and soft vowel within each series. This requires a slight adjustment of the vocal cords to the rate of air flow. This exercise can be varied by having him accent every third vowel as well as having him use other patterns of accent. It can be done on a series containing a single vowel and proceed to varying the vowel within a series.

6. Have the child alternate a whisper and vocalization in a series of vowels. This is done on a single exhalation. The sounds are produced rapidly and intensity held constant. The air flow is stopped between sounds with the child inhaling only between series. He should begin with only four syllables in a series.

7. The child is asked to produce /hɑ/ and /ɑ/ alternately. He should not prolong or emphasize the /h/. He can proceed to /u/ and /i/ in the same manner, and then go on to alternating the vowels in a single series. As the exercises are perfected and breathiness diminishes, more complex combinations of vowels and consonants can be used. The child should use phrases at a normal speech rate and be able to maintain desirable voice quality.

Goal 5. Rate and Rhythm

Rate and rhythm of speaking need special attention in the hearing-impaired child. Some children speak with excessively slow rate and inappropriate rhythm. A child's slow rate of speaking may be related to lack of breath control. For example, he may need to take a breath every few words and not have enough breath to finish a phrase. The speech clinician should plan a program of improvement. Our method of modifying rate using the rate chart (Fig. 33) is useful for most children with hearing losses. Hudgins' (12) fifth and sixth exercises for breathiness, using patterns of accented and unaccented vowels and nonsense syllables, are useful in correcting rate and rhythm problems. With some children it is sufficient to make a simple, direct request for more rapid rate and to urge the child to maintain a rhythmic flow of speech if he lags. It may be necessary to begin this program by coordinating gross bodily movements with music (26, pp. 19/3–12). These are then applied to the rate and rhythm of speaking. All children with impaired hearing should do a great deal of carefully supervised group singing, with emphasis on using correct rate, rhythm, and pitch. Haycock (11, p. 267) recommended the clinician beat time as the child speaks by using a wide swing of the arm for an accented syllable or word and a light downward movement of the hand for the unaccented. In advanced work, one continuous swing of the arm might be used for an entire short sentence.

The relationship of speech rate to intelligibility in a group of deaf subjects was studied by Tato and Arcella (23). They measured habitual speech rates on familiar written passages. The average rate was 0.47 sec a syllable and the range was from 0.30 to 0.76. A comparable group of hearing children averaged 0.20 sec and ranged from 0.17 to 0.27 sec. After a month's training the deaf subjects' rate was reduced to 0.28 sec a syllable and ranged from 0.20 to 0.42, which was close to the rate for normal children. The intelligibility of the deaf group was judged by a group of listeners to improve markedly in 27 % of the cases, to show no significant change in 36 %, and to deteriorate markedly in the other 37 %. Thus, it appears only selected hearing-impaired children can improve intelligibility by increasing the rate of speaking. Before increasing rate in a hearing-impaired child, the speech clinician should check the effect of increased rate on intelligibility. Only those children who have improved intelligibility as a result of increased rate should be instructed to maintain the increased rate habitually.

Goal 6. Elimination or Modification of Vocal Abuse

Many hearing-impaired children use various forms of vocal abuse. Some of these abuses occur during play and sports activity as part of the pattern of usual exuberance and enthusiasm exhibited by all participants. Other vocal abuses may occur as a child forces phonation in an attempt to be understood. If the laryngeal tone is hoarse and if the analysis of vocal abuse reveals any abuses being used excessively and to a severe degree, the clinician should develop a program of elimination or modification. Positive laryngeal findings such as vocal nodules definitely indicate the necessity for such a program. In the absence of pathology a program of elimination or modification of vocal abuse serves as a preventive measure for developing pathology. The program for vocal abuse in Chapter 5, adapted to the needs of the hearing-impaired child, should be followed.

This chapter can be summarized by describing voice therapy procedures used with a 7-year-old boy. Jim had an unaided speech reception threshold of 80 dB and aided speech reception of 45 dB (ISO, 1964). His habitual pitch was too high and uncontrolled and his laryngeal tone was breathy. He habitually talked too loud and did much uncontrolled shouting. He used abrupt glottal attacks and his rate of speaking was too slow.

Therapy was initiated with work on pitch, and other problems were approached after the first session. Listening training for pitch began with awareness of differences in others. The clinician read a story using a very high pitch intermittently on words. Jim signalled by pressing a button which activated a red light each time he heard the high pitch. When he learned accurately and reliably to recognize the occurrence of high pitch in the clinician's voice, he was ready to do gross discrimination of differences. He was given the task of recognizing the extremes of very high pitch and very low pitch in the clinician's voice. He pushed the appropriate button on a switch panel—red for too high and yellow for too low. When he could accurately discriminate gross pitch differences he then went on to fine discrimination of differences. He was taught to recognize each level of pitch as the clinician used three levels ranging through very low, correct, and very high. He used the switch panel to activate appropriate lights. A green light was added to indicate correct pitch level.

After Jim had completed the program of listening to others he was ready to apply these procedures to the pitch of his own voice. His own recordings were used to develop awareness of the high pitch and to develop gross and fine discrimination of pitch levels in his voice. He was then ready to be taught conscious control of pitch. Jim was first asked to speak words on two pitch levels: too high and correct. When he had gained voluntary control over these two levels he then produced at will a very high pitch and a very low pitch. Next he produced three levels of pitch, high, middle, and low, selecting the middle one as the correct pitch level for his own use. After practicing the correct pitch level Jim began transfer of his new pitch into habitual use. This was done in a limited way at first with the clinician. Then outside assignments were added until he used adequate voice pitch in all situations.

The elimination of the abrupt glottal attack was incorporated into the the ongoing program. Jim was taught the kinesthetic cues of abrupt, explosive vocalization contrasting these to the sensations felt during an easy initiation. Jim was taught to shout in an easier, effortless way following the program suggested by Uris (24) (Chapter 5). We worked on increasing rate and decreasing breathiness while we worked on pitch. As a result of the therapy program, Jim gained control over his use of loudness and pitch and eliminated the vocal abuses. He had a more pleasant voice with improved quality. His rate of speaking was normal and his speech intelligibility had improved.

Each child with a hearing loss may need to work toward a different combination of goals. He may need to be shown how to use balanced resonance without excessive hypernasality or hyponasality for a more pleasant voice. A correct habitual pitch level with appropriate inflections is necessary. The loudness of voice may need adjustment to an appropriate level. A clear laryngeal tone free from harshness, hoarseness, or breathiness is desirable. Teaching correct rate and rhythm of speaking may make speech more intelligible. Eliminating or modifying vocal abuse assures better voice hygiene. Often several parameters are simultaneously approached for a unified program of voice improvement. This program must be adapted to each child's needs and his hearing ability and coordinated with the total auditory and speech program.

REFERENCES

1. Arnold, G. E. Physiology and pathology of speech and language. In R. Luchsinger and G. E. Arnold. *Voice—speech—language. Clinical communicology: Its physiology and pathology.* Belmont: Wadsworth Publishing Company, 1965.
2. Berg, F. S. Educational audiology. In F. S. Berg and S. G. Fletcher (Editors), *The hard of hearing child. Clinical and educational management.* New York: Grune and Stratton, 1970.
3. Berry, M. F., and Eisenson, J. *Speech disorders. Principles and practices of therapy.* New York: Appleton-Century-Crofts, Inc., 1956.
4. Boone, D. R. Modification of the voices of deaf children. *Volta Rev.,* **68,** 1966, 686–692.
5. Engleberg, M. Correction of falsetto voice in a deaf adult. *J. Speech Hearing Dis.,* **27,** 1962, 162–164.
6. Ermovick, D. A. A spectrographic analysis comparing connected speech of deaf subjects and hearing subjects. Unpublished master's thesis, University of Kansas, 1965.

7. Froeschels, E. Hygiene of the voice. *Arch. Otolaryng. (Chicago)*, **38**, 1943, 122–130.
8. Froeschels, E. Chewing method as therapy. *Arch. Otolaryng. (Chicago)*, **56**, 1952, 427–432.
9. Fuller, C. W. Differential diagnosis. In F. S. Berg and S. G. Fletcher (Editors), *The hard of hearing child. Clinical and educational management.* New York: Grune and Stratton, 1970.
10. Greene, M. C. L. *The voice and its disorders.* Ed. 2. New York: Macmillan Company, 1957.
11. Haycock, G. S. *The teaching of speech.* Stoke-on-Trent, England: Hill and Ainsworth, Ltd., 1933. Reprintings by Volta Bureau, Washington, D. C.
12. Hudgins, C. V. Voice production and breath control in the speech of the deaf. *Amer. Ann. Deaf*, **82**, 1937, 338–363.
13. Irwin, R. B. *Speech and hearing therapy. Clinical and educational principles and practices.* Pittsburgh: Stanwix House, 1965.
14. Meckfessel, A. L. A comparison between vocal characteristics of deaf and normal hearing individuals. Unpublished master's thesis, University of Kansas, 1965.
15. Miller, E. A public school program for hard of hearing children. *J. Speech Hearing Dis.*, **13**, 1948, 256–259.
16. Miller, J. Speech and the preschool child. *Volta Rev.*, **62**, 1960, 315–317.
17. New, M. C. Speech suggestions for the hard of hearing. *Hearing News*, **13**, March, 1945.
18. Pollack, D. *Educational audiology for the limited hearing infant.* Springfield, Ill.: Charles C Thomas, 1970.
19. Presto, M. An experiment in voice control. *Volta Rev.*, **45**, 1943, 490–493.
20. Sanders, D. A. *Aural rehabilitation.* Englewood Cliffs: Prentice-Hall, Inc., 1971.
21. Silverman, S. R., and Davis, H. Hard-of-hearing children. In H. Davis and S. R. Silverman (Editors), *Hearing and deafness.* Ed. 3. New York: Holt, Rinehart and Winston, 1970.
22. Streng, A., Fitch, W. J., Hedgecock, L. D., Phillips, J. W., and Carrell, J. A. *Hearing therapy for children.* Ed. 2. New York: Grune and Stratton, 1958.
23. Tato, J. M., and Arcella, A. I. La inteligibilidad en funcion della velocidad de la palabra hablada en los sordos desmutizados. *Acta Otorinolaring. Iber. Amer.*, **23**, 1962, 551–560. Cited by Quigley, S. P. Language research in countries other than the United States. *Volta Rev.*, **68**, 1966, 68–83.
24. Uris, D. Teen talk. *Todays Speech*, **10**, 1962, 15–16.
25. Van Riper, C. Binaural speech therapy. *J. Speech Hearing Dis.*, **24**, 1959, 62–63.
26. Van Uden, A. A sound perceptive method. In Sir A. Ewing (Editor), *The modern educational treatment of deafness.* Manchester: University Press, 1960.
27. Wilson, D. K. Voice problems of hearing-impaired children. In *Proceedings of international congress on education of deaf, Stockholm, 1970.* Saga/Svensk Lararetidnings, Forlags AB, in press.

INDEX